To The Reader

This book is presented as part of the religious literature and works of Scientology® Founder, L. Ron Hubbard. It is a record of Mr. Hubbard's observations and research into the nature of man and each individual's capabilities as a spiritual being, and is not a statement of claims made by the author, publisher or any Church of Scientology.

Scientology is defined as the study and handling of the spirit in relationship to itself, universes and other life. Thus, the mission of the Church of Scientology is a simple one: to help the individual regain his true nature, as a spiritual being, and thereby attain an awareness of his relationship with his fellow man and the universe. Therein lies the path to personal integrity, trust, enlightenment and spiritual freedom itself.

Scientology and its forerunner and substudy, Dianetics, as practiced by the Church, address only the "thetan" (spirit), which is senior to the body, and its relationship to and effects on the body. While the Church is free, as all churches are, to engage in spiritual healing, its primary goal is increased spiritual awareness for all. For this reason, neither Scientology nor Dianetics is offered as, nor professes to be physical healing, nor is any claim made to that effect. Therefore, the Purification Program and the vitamin and mineral regimens described in this book cannot be construed as a recommendation of medical treatment or medication. They are not professed or offered as physical healing, nor is any claim made to that effect.

The Church does not accept individuals who desire treatment of physical or mental illness but, instead, requires a competent medical examination for physical conditions, by qualified specialists before addressing their spiritual cause. No individual should undertake the Purification Program or any of its regimens without first consulting and obtaining the informed approval of a qualified, licensed medical practitioner.

The Hubbard® Electrometer, or E-Meter, is a religious artifact used in the Church. The E-Meter, by itself, does nothing and is only used by ministers and ministers-in-training, qualified in its use, to help parishioners locate the source of spiritual travail.

The attainment of the benefits and goals of the Scientology religion requires each individual's dedicated participation, as only through one's own efforts can they be achieved.

We hope reading this book is only one step of a personal voyage of discovery into this new and vital world religion.

Narconon International and its affiliated Narconon Centers around the world constitute a drug rehabilitation network utilizing a secular program derived from the detoxification methods found in the Purification Program. Any interested reader can contact one of the Narconon Centers for further information concerning their program and use of detoxification for drug rehabilitation purposes.

This Book Belongs To

_____

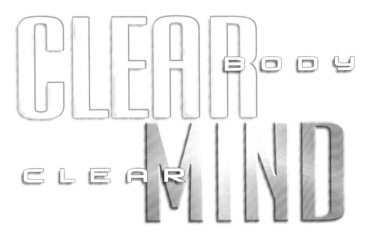

CLEAR BODY CLEAR MIND

THE EFFECTIVE PURIFICATION PROGRAM

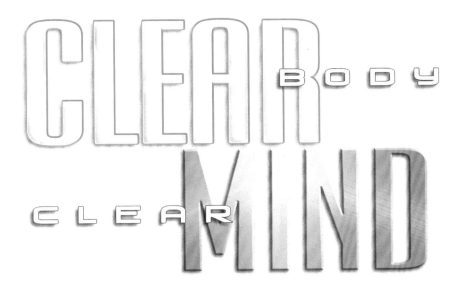

CLEAR BODY CLEAR MIND

THE EFFECTIVE PURIFICATION PROGRAM

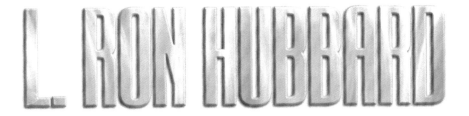

L. RON HUBBARD

Bridge Publications, Inc.™

A
HUBBARD®
PUBLICATION

Bridge Publications, Inc.
5600 E. Olympic Boulevard
Commerce, California 90022

ISBN 978-1-4572-2793-6

Clear Body, Clear Mind—English

Important Note

In reading this book, be very certain you never go past a word you do not fully understand. The only reason a person gives up a study or becomes confused or unable to learn is because he or she has gone past a word that was not understood.

The confusion or inability to grasp or learn comes AFTER a word the person did not have defined and understood. It may not only be the new and unusual words you have to look up. Some commonly used words can often be misdefined and so cause confusion.

This datum about not going past an undefined word is the most important fact in the whole subject of study. Every subject you have taken up and abandoned had its words which you failed to get defined.

Therefore, in studying this book be very, very certain you never go past a word you do not fully understand. If the material becomes confusing or you can't seem to grasp it, there will be a word just earlier that you have not understood. Don't go any further, but go back to BEFORE you got into trouble, find the misunderstood word and get it defined.

Glossary

To aid reader comprehension, L. Ron Hubbard directed the editors to provide a glossary. This is included in the Appendix, *Editor's Glossary of Words, Terms and Phrases*. Words sometimes have several meanings. The *Editor's Glossary* only contains the definitions of words as they are used in this text. Other definitions can be found in standard language or Dianetics and Scientology dictionaries.

If you find any other words you do not know, look them up in a good dictionary.

$\mathcal{T}$HE PURIFICATION PROGRAM does not supplant technology I developed earlier that is now in use, especially in Narconon drug rehabilitation centers, for handling persons currently on drugs and apt to experience withdrawal symptoms when taken off them. The Purification Program would be begun only after such technology had been applied.

No medicines or drugs are used on the Purification Program. The only dosages recommended are those classified as food. No medical recommendations or claims are made for the program. The only claim is future spiritual improvement.

The program demands rigid adherence to the guidelines researched and established for its use. No individual should undertake this action on his own.

The data contained herein is a record of research and results noted. It cannot be construed as a recommendation for medical treatment or medication and it is undertaken or delivered by any individual on his own responsibility.

I have never received any percentage of fees for administering this program. My development of it is a contribution and gift to my friends.

L. RON HUBBARD

CONTENTS

$\mathcal{I}$NTRODUCTION

$\mathcal{T}$HE PLANET HAS hit a barrier that prevents any widespread social progress: drugs and other toxic substances.

These can put people into a condition that not only prohibits and destroys physical health, but which can prevent any stable advancement in mental or spiritual well-being.

My major work since the late 1930s has consisted of research into the nature and spirit of Man. The resultant discoveries made possible the development of specific technologies to assist Man to find out who he is and where he is going. They have opened the door to levels of mental achievement and spiritual freedom that many have dreamed of throughout the centuries but rarely believed attainable.

Such studies could not advance by ignoring Man's concern with his physical problems. Thus some of my earliest research was carried out in the fields of nutrition, vitamin therapy, the effects of radiation, drugs and other related factors.

Since the early '50s, I have known that it was a mistake to expect any stable personal improvement in someone who has been on drugs until the effects of the drugs have been handled. If the person is still on drugs, attempts to help him will have little lasting effect. The drugs trap him.

The problem was not a widespread one in 1950, but by 1960 drug use had become far more common. And as the '60s progressed, the explosion of drug usage became planetwide.

Given the increasing devastation wrought by drugs, an immediate resolution was required. So I embarked upon more extensive research into the effects of drugs on the body, mind and spirit.

The result was the Purification Program.

The program is based on data gathered in a pilot program and on a number of fundamental principles discovered in my decades of study of Man's ability to improve his condition. Since its release in 1979, reports of resounding benefits from its precise application have been received, exceeding even the original expectations.

This book has been written, therefore, in response to numerous requests that the theory and technology of the Purification Program be published broadly. It includes, in brief, a chronicle of my research, theories and discoveries that form the basis for the program.

If the Purification Program can be used to salvage even a part of a civilization sick from the onslaught of drugs and other toxic substances, then perhaps there is hope for *all* of that civilization.

PART ONE

The Breakthrough of the Purification Program

CLEAR BODY, CLEAR MIND

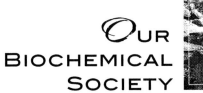
Our Biochemical Society

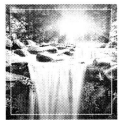

Our Biochemical Society

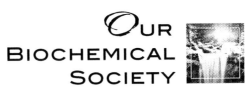

*W*E LIVE IN a chemical-oriented society.

One would be hard put to find someone in the present-day civilization who is not affected by this fact. Every day the vast majority of the public is subjected to the intake of food preservatives and other chemical poisons, including atmospheric poisons and pesticides. Added to this are the pain pills, tranquilizers, psychiatric and other medical drugs prescribed by doctors. Additionally the widespread use of marijuana, LSD, cocaine and other street drugs contribute heavily to the scene.

These factors are *all* part of the biochemical problem.

BIOCHEMICAL means the interaction of life forms and chemical substances.

BIO- means life, of living things; from the Greek *bios,* life or way of life.

CHEMICAL means of or having to do with chemicals. Chemicals are substances, simple or complex, that are the building blocks of matter.

The human body is composed of certain exact chemicals and chemical compounds, with complex chemical processes going on continuously within it. Some substances, such as nutrients, air and water, are vital to the continuation of these processes and for maintaining the body's health. Other substances are relatively neutral when entered into the body, causing neither benefit nor damage. Still other substances can wreak havoc, blocking or perverting body functions and making the body ill or even killing it.

TOXIC SUBSTANCES, which fall into this last category, are those that upset the body's normal chemical balance or interfere with its processes. The term is used to describe drugs, chemicals or any substance shown to be poisonous or harmful to an organism. The word *toxic* itself comes from the Greek word *toxikon,* which originally meant a poison in which arrows were dipped.

DETOXIFICATION would be the action of removing a poison or a poisonous effect from something, such as from one's body.

Toxins in Abundance

An enormous volume of material has been written on the subject of toxic substances, their reported effects and the prospects for their handling. Examples abound in publications and news reports.

The current environment is permeated with life-hostile elements. Drugs, radioactive wastes, pollutants and chemical agents of all types are not only everywhere, but are becoming even more prevalent as time goes on. In fact, they are so commonplace they are almost impossible to avoid.

For example, some of the things put in canned vegetables or soup could be considered toxic. They are preservatives and the action of a preservative is to impede decay. Yet digestion and cellular action are based on decay. In other words, those things might be great for the manufacturer, as they preserve the product, *but* they could be very bad for the consumer. It is not that I am on a food faddism kick or a kick against preservatives. The point is that Man is surrounded by toxins.

This example alone of preservatives in foods illustrates the degree to which one can encounter toxic substances in daily living.

But combine that with the enemies of various countries using widespread drug addiction as a defeatist mechanism and nations vying with each other in the manufacture and testing of nuclear weapons (and so increasing the amount of radioactive material free in the environment). Then add the ready availability of painkillers and sedatives, the increased use of industrial and agricultural chemicals, and toxic substances developed for chemical warfare. In short (and putting it bluntly), this society, at this time, is riddled with toxic substances.

Certain data regarding those substances that pose a threat to individuals and to society at large will bring the biochemical situation more clearly into focus. It is to this situation that the Purification Program is addressed.

Drugs

Drugs are essentially poisons. The degree to which they are taken determines the effect. A small amount acts as a stimulant (increases activity). A greater amount acts as a sedative (suppresses activity). A larger amount acts as a poison and can kill one dead.

This is true of any drug and each has a different amount at which it gives those results. Caffeine is a drug, so coffee is an example. One hundred cups of coffee would probably kill a person. Ten cups would probably put him to sleep. Two or three cups stimulates. This is a very common drug. It is not very harmful, as it takes so much of it to have an effect. So it is known as a stimulant.

Arsenic is a known poison. Yet a tiny amount of arsenic is a stimulant, a larger dose puts one to sleep and a few grains kill.

Street Drugs

The drug scene is planetwide and swimming in blood and human misery.

Research demonstrates that the single most destructive element present in our current culture is drugs.

The acceleration of widespread use of drugs such as LSD, heroin, cocaine, marijuana and the litany of new street drugs all play a part in our debilitated society. Even schoolchildren are shoved on to drugs. And children of drug-taking mothers are born as druggies.

Reportedly some of these drugs can cause brain and nerve damage. Marijuana, for example, so favored by college students, who are supposed to be getting bright today so they can be the executives of tomorrow, is reported capable of causing brain atrophy.

Research even established that there is such a thing as a "drug personality." It is artificial and is created by drugs. Drugs can apparently change the attitude of persons from their original personality to one secretly harboring hostilities and hatreds they do not permit to show on the surface. While this may not hold true in all cases, it does establish a link between drugs and increasing difficulties with crime, failing productivity and the modern breakdown of social and industrial culture.

The devastating physiological effects of drugs are the subject of newspaper headlines routinely. That they also result in a breakdown of mental alertness and ethical fiber is all too obvious.

But vicious and damaging though they are, street drugs are actually only one part of the biochemical problem.

Medical and Psychiatric Drugs

Medical and, most particularly, the long list of psychiatric drugs (Ritalin, Valium, Thorazine and lithium, to name a few) can be every bit as damaging as street drugs. The prevalence of these currently in common use would be quite amazing to one unfamiliar with the problem.

Sedatives are often administered as though they were a panacea for all ills. As early as 1951, many persons had become so accustomed to their daily dosage of sleeping pills or painkillers that they did not consider their "little pills" as drugs.

Too often the attitude is "If I can't find the cause of the pain, at least I'll deaden it." In the case of one who is mentally ill, this might read, "If he can't be made rational, at least he can be made quiet."

Unfortunately it is not recognized that a person whose pain has been deadened by a sedative has himself been deadened by the same drug and is much nearer the ultimate pain of death. It should be obvious that the quietest people in the world are the dead.

Alcohol

Alcohol is not a mind-altering drug, but it is a biochemical-altering drug. Alcohol doesn't do anything to the mind; it does something to the nerves. By quickly and rapidly soaking up all the vitamin B_1

in the body, it makes the nerves incapable of functioning properly. Therefore a person can't coordinate his body. Alcohol in small quantities is a stimulant and in large quantities is a depressant.

The definition of *alcoholics* is individuals who can't have just *one* drink. If they have one drink, they have to have another. They are addicted. One of the factors is they have to have a full glass in front of them. If it gets empty, it has to be refilled.

Alcoholics are in a state of total, unrelenting hostility toward everything around them. They will do people in without even mentioning it.

Alcohol is a drug. The degree of alcohol consumption (quantity and frequency) determines whether an individual should be considered a heavy user.

Commercial Processes and Products

In recent years much research has been done on the potential toxic effects of many of the substances commonly used in various commercial processes and products and to what extent they may find their way into the bodies of this planet's inhabitants. Following are a few examples of what this research is bringing to light.

INDUSTRIAL CHEMICALS

Under this heading exist the tens of thousands of chemicals used in manufacturing. Not all such chemicals are toxic, of course. But workers in factories that produce or use such things as pesticides, petroleum products, plastics, detergents and cleaning chemicals, solvents, plated metals, preservatives, drugs, asbestos products, fertilizers, some cosmetics, perfumes, paints, dyes, electrical equipment or any radioactive materials can be exposed, often for extended periods, to toxic materials. Of course, the consumer can be exposed to residual amounts of such chemicals when they use these products.

Agricultural Chemicals

Pesticides are the most obvious of the toxic substances to which workers in agricultural activities could be exposed. These include insecticides (insect-killing chemicals), herbicides (chemicals to kill unwanted plants, such as weeds) and man-made fertilizers.

Under the heading of herbicides come several that contain a substance called "dioxin," known to be a highly toxic chemical even in amounts almost too small to detect in the body.

Contact with chemicals used in agriculture can occur in a number of ways. The chemical can be carried on or in the plant itself and so eaten. It can be carried on the wind and breathed in directly by those living or working in agricultural areas. It can even be carried into drinking-water supplies.

Food, Food Additives and Preservatives

There are substances added to some commercially processed foods that are meant to "enhance" color or flavor or, as mentioned previously, to keep the food from spoiling. Also becoming more common are various artificial sweeteners used in "diet" soft drinks and other commercially packaged foods. From research on these "enhancers" and "sweeteners" and "preservers," it appears that many of them are quite toxic. The whole subject of food additives and preservatives has become a matter of concern to many people.

There is another side to this matter of food. Research findings point to the possibility that rancid oils are a health hazard of a magnitude not previously suspected. Oils used in cooking or commercial processing of foods, where they are not fresh, pure and free of rancidity, have been linked, by researchers, with digestive and muscular ills and even cancer.

PERFUMES AND FRAGRANCES

Use of perfumes and fragrances in all sorts of products has become more and more prevalent in recent years. Everything from clothing and laundry detergent, to facial tissue and magazine advertisements, has fragrance added to it. That fragrance is usually a cheap chemical derivative, an extract of coal tar that probably costs about 10 cents for a 50-gallon drum. Findings seem to bear out that these chemicals, floating about in the local supermarket as "fragrances," are actually toxic and can end up in the food products sold there. Ingesting these chemicals is clearly no aid to digestion.

Radiation

You've no doubt seen in the news that contact with radiation can occur through exposure to nuclear weapons tests (or the radioactive particles they can release into the atmosphere), to nuclear wastes or to some manufacturing processes that use radioactive materials. Further, the increased use of atomic power for electrical supply, without developing proper technology and safeguards in its use, poses a nonmilitary threat. And the deterioration of the upper atmosphere of the planet by pollutants year by year lets more and more solar radiation through to the planetary surface.

In other words, there are many ways one can be exposed to radiation. It's all over the atmosphere and always has been. There is just more of it now.

Sun worshipers, sunbathers, those who make a career of baking themselves in the sun year after year, expose themselves to radiation. What is the Sun but a ball of radiation? No better example of radiation can be found anywhere than our own Sun. Therefore a sunburn *is* a burn, but not a burn that occurs simply from excessive heat: it is a radiation burn. A certain amount of sunlight is probably essential to the good health of the human body. It is excessive exposure we are talking about here. Even when one does not burn, per se, with extensive daily exposure over long periods of time, one is subjected to the cumulative effects of radiation.

X-rays also expose one to radiation. They are fully as deadly as atomic fission. X-ray does not bring about the big bang; you don't get a tremendous explosion and no town left. But it does, X-ray by X-ray, bring about a condition of high count in the individual so that if one gets a little bit more X-ray or fallout, one is liable to become ill. A repeated, continuous application of X-ray to a person can bring about anything and everything that atomic fission brings about in its pollution of the atmosphere.

Where there is a radioactive atmosphere, there is also a declining health rate. The more people are exposed to radiation, the less resistance they have and the more effect the radiation has on them. In other words, a buildup occurs in the body, over time, from any of the sources described above. As radiation is cumulative, it follows, then, that this compounds the biochemical problem and presents a barrier of magnitude.

An Answer to the Biochemical World

In light of all of the above, the Purification Program is a proffered answer to this biochemical problem. In a society as pervaded with drugs and toxic materials as this one has become, handling accumulations of such materials should be a point of great interest.

The logical questions regarding any procedure that might handle such accumulations would be "Does it work?" "Does it get *results?*"

These questions are answered by practical experience and through an understanding of the basic discoveries that brought about a procedure to free the individual from the harmful effects of toxic substances.

~

THE DEVELOPMENT OF THE PURIFICATION PROGRAM

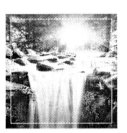

The Development of the Purification Program

*W*ITH THE EXPLOSION of the drug problem in the 1960s, when the use of illicit street drugs and their ravaging effects had become a dominant factor among society's ills, I developed a set of procedures called the Drug Rundown. The Drug Rundown deals directly with the mental effect of drugs that can affect an individual adversely. The rundown frees attention from past drug incidents so people are more able to deal with life and better able to control themselves and the things in their surroundings. This rundown remains in use today as the final resolution to any drug handling.

However, in the 1970s, it became apparent that underlying factors may need to be handled prior to doing this rundown. Working with individuals who had been drug users, in a study of their physical symptoms and behavioral patterns, I made a startling discovery:

PEOPLE WHO HAD BEEN ON LSD AT SOME EARLIER TIME APPEARED TO RELAPSE AND ACT AS IF THEY HAD JUST TAKEN MORE LSD.

As it has been stated that it takes only one millionth of an ounce of LSD to produce a drugged condition and because LSD is basically wheat rust, which simply cuts off the circulation, my original thinking on this was that LSD must remain in the body.

The most likely place for a toxic substance to lock up is in the body's fatty tissue. It has been said that in middle age, the body's ability to break down fat decreases. So here we have, apparently, a situation of toxic substances locked up in fatty tissue and the fatty tissue is not being broken down. As a result, such toxic substances can accumulate.

In other words:

LSD APPARENTLY STAYS IN THE SYSTEM, LODGING IN THE TISSUES, MAINLY THE FATTY TISSUES OF THE BODY, AND IS LIABLE TO GO INTO ACTION AGAIN, GIVING THE PERSON UNPREDICTABLE "TRIPS" EVEN YEARS AFTER THE PERSON HAS COME OFF LSD.

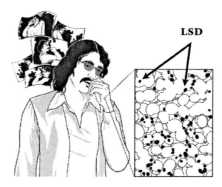

LSD apparently stays in the system, lodging in the tissues, mainly the fatty tissues of the body...

LSD

1968

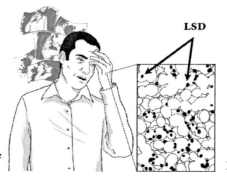

...and is liable to go into action again, giving the person unpredictable "trips" even years after the person has come off LSD.

LSD

1980

Thus the behavior, actions and responsibility level of those who had taken LSD were unpredictable! Not to mention that these "flashbacks" could be quite fatal while driving or even walking around.

What was the answer to these cases?

No known method existed for ridding the body of these minute drug deposits that, locked as they were in the tissues, were not totally dispelled in the normal processes of elimination.

The answer obviously did not lie in attempting to handle this with more drugs or biochemicals, which would only compound the situation. But could a method be evolved to dislodge and flush these deposits out, thereby freeing the person for full rehabilitation physically as well as mentally and spiritually?

The Original "Sweat Program"

In 1977, I developed and released a regimen called the "Sweat Program." It operated on the premise that the negative factors observed might be reversed if there were a means of getting LSD deposits out of the system and that the most logical method to accomplish that would be to sweat them out.

My theory was borne out in practice as persons on the program experienced the apparent exudation of LSD and newly felt the effects of the drug. But it wasn't just LSD that was coming out: they reported smelling or tasting or feeling the effects of a host of other street drugs and chemicals, the same ones they had consumed or were exposed to years earlier.

They were also experiencing, in mild form, some of the sensations of old sunburns, past illnesses and injuries and other past physical and emotional conditions.

Therefore it appeared that:

> NOT ONLY LSD, BUT OTHER CHEMICAL POISONS AND TOXINS,
> PRESERVATIVES, PESTICIDES, ETC., AS WELL AS MEDICINAL
> DRUGS AND THE LONG LIST OF STREET DRUGS (HEROIN,
> MARIJUANA, COCAINE, ETC.), CAN LODGE IN THE TISSUES
> AND REMAIN IN THE BODY FOR YEARS.

> EVEN MEDICINAL DRUGS SUCH AS DIET PILLS, CODEINE,
> NOVOCAIN AND OTHERS, AS WELL AS PSYCHIATRIC DRUGS,
> CAN BE REACTIVATED YEARS AFTER THEY WERE TAKEN AND
> SUPPOSEDLY HAD BEEN ELIMINATED FROM THE BODY.

Thus it seemed that any or all of these hostile biochemical substances could get caught in the tissues and their accumulation probably disarranged the biochemistry and fluid balance of the body.

This was my early thinking on the subject. It was now being borne out by further research as more and more manifestations occurred. (It has also since been borne out by clinical tests and by medical autopsies that have found deposits of certain drugs embedded in body tissues.)

Moreover, as research continued with those on the Sweat Program, all indicators were that these substances were being flushed out as people progressed on the program. And these same individuals were reporting that they felt a new vigor, a renewed vitality and interest in life.

The Sweat Program was a lengthy process, however, taking months to complete. A refinement and speed-up was needed and so I developed the Purification Program.

Elements of the Purification Program

The Purification Program is a tightly supervised regimen that includes the following elements:

1. Exercise (running).
2. Sauna sweat-out.
3. Nutrition, including vitamins, minerals, etc., as well as oil intake.
4. A properly ordered personal schedule.

Participants run to get the blood circulating deeper into the tissues where toxic residuals are lodged and thus to loosen and release the accumulated harmful deposits and get them moving.

It is very important, then, that the running be immediately followed by sweating in the sauna to flush out these dislodged accumulations.

While supplementing one's regular diet with plenty of fresh vegetables, one also takes an exact regimen of vitamins, minerals and extra quantities of oil. The recommended vitamin dosages are gradiently increased over the course of the program. (By *gradiently* is meant a gradual approach to something, taken step by step: in this case, a gradual increase of vitamins.) This regimen is not only a vital factor in helping the body flush out toxins, it also repairs and rebuilds areas affected by drugs and other toxic residuals.

A proper schedule with enough rest is mandatory because the body undergoes change and repair throughout the program.

These actions, carried out on a very stringently monitored basis, apparently accomplish a detoxification of the entire system, to the renewed health and vigor of the individual.

Mental and Spiritual Aspects

There is, however, a more in-depth and comprehensive view to be taken of the entire process, including the mental and spiritual aspects of the program. For beyond any physical damage they may cause, many drugs—marijuana, peyote, morphine, heroin, to name but a few—have another liability: they directly affect the person's mind. As one example, LSD, originally designed for psychiatric use, can reportedly make schizophrenics out of normal people.

But to better understand these mental effects of drugs, it is necessary to know something about what the mind is.

As people go through life, their minds record pictures of everything they perceive, moment by moment, twenty-four hours a day. These *mental image pictures* are three-dimensional color pictures that contain all perceptions—all that the individual has seen, heard, felt, smelled, tasted and experienced.

The consecutive record of mental image pictures that accumulates through a person's life is called the *time track*. It is very exactly dated. Ordinarily one's time track is made up of the recorded moment-to-moment events experienced as one moves through life. However, a person who has taken drugs, in addition to the physical factors involved, retains mental image pictures of those drugs and their effects. In other words, their time track for that period is not made up of present time events only. Instead it is jumbled: their mental records and perceptions are distorted and tangled up, combining actual events, imagination and pictures from incidents in the past.

For example, let us say at some point in time an individual took LSD at an outdoor rock concert on a hot summer day. Let us further suppose that the person experienced a number of severe side effects while under the influence of the drug. These included higher body temperature, increased heart rate, rapid mood swings and nausea set off by the smell of cigarette smoke. Sometime during the day he was separated from his friends, panicked and was overcome with anxiety. He also suffered hallucinations, specifically "hearing" colors and "seeing" sounds. This individual would have mental image pictures of everything connected to that drug incident, including imagination and the hallucinations caused by the LSD. And those pictures could unexpectedly affect him at a later time.

Sometime in the future, if this person's environment were to contain enough similarities to that past LSD incident, the incident could be restimulated (reactivated or stimulated again). For example, he might be outside on a hot day and hear loud music playing. Someone nearby might light a cigarette and blow the smoke in his direction. These factors are enough to set off the drug-induced experiences of that day at the concert. His heart might suddenly begin racing and he might feel nauseous. He might also become overwhelmed with anxiety for no apparent reason. And then again, he might experience the same type of hallucinations involving sight and sound. In other words, without taking any more of the drug, the mental images could be restimulated and he could re-experience that drug incident.

On the other hand, there is the matter of drug residuals. Residues from the LSD he took that day at the concert remain trapped in his body. Even years later, some of those LSD crystals could suddenly become dislodged from fatty tissue and release back into his system. In so doing, the drug would be activated and send him on a new "trip," as if he had just taken more LSD.

Therefore, on the Purification Program, two factors must be considered:

1. The actual drugs and toxic residuals in the body.
2. The mental image pictures of the drugs and the mental image pictures of one's experiences with these drugs.

These two factors are hung up, one playing against the other, in perfect balance. What the person is feeling is the two conditions: the actual presence of the drug residuals and the mental image pictures relating to them.

The Purification Program handles one of these factors, the accumulated toxic residuals. And this fixes the person up so that the other factor, the mental image pictures, are no longer restimulative or in constant restimulation. It is as simple as that.

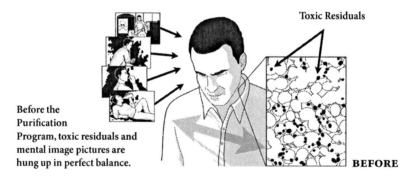

Toxic Residuals

Before the Purification Program, toxic residuals and mental image pictures are hung up in perfect balance.

BEFORE

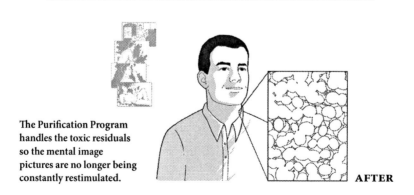

The Purification Program handles the toxic residuals so the mental image pictures are no longer being constantly restimulated.

AFTER

What happens on the Purification Program, among other things, is an upset of this perfect balance. Suddenly the balance and cross-reaction are gone. The harmful and restimulative chemical residues are flushed out and gone. This does not, however, mean the mental image pictures are gone. But they are no longer in restimulation and they are not being reinforced by the presence of drug residuals.

By breaking up the balance between these two factors and handling the toxic residuals on the Purification Program, we remove elements destructive to the individual's physical health and free him for mental and spiritual gain. In other words, the person is now in a state where he can pursue betterment of his own perceptions and abilities.

The Purification Program: A "Long-range Detoxification" Program

Even someone off drugs for years still has "blank periods." Drugs can injure a person's ability to concentrate, to work and to learn. Drug residues can stop any mental help. They also stop a person's life!

While the Purification Program originally addressed the handling of accumulated drugs in the system, it also appears to flush out many other toxic substances accumulated by the body.

These substances must be eliminated if one is to get stable mental and spiritual gain. The operating rule is that mental actions and even biophysical actions (methods of improving the person's ability to handle one's body and environment) do not work in the presence of life-hostile elements.

So, in rehabilitating an individual, only when we have accomplished a biochemical handling can we then go on to the next step, the biophysical handling (improving the person's awareness of the environment and ability to face the present) and then on to further mental and spiritual improvement.

My development of a program to handle drugs, along with drug and chemical deposits in the body, was based on the fact that successful rehabilitation of an individual can only be accomplished in the sequence outlined above. When one tries to move these steps around and put them out of sequence, one gets losses. Moreover, a full rehabilitation requires all steps to be done.

Apparent gain occurs by cleaning up the body and can be seen as an end-all in itself, though that was not the original motivation. In view of what it evidently accomplishes, however, the Purification Program might be termed a long-range detoxification program. But it should be identified as itself, since it is unique among detoxification programs, both in its procedure and reported results. To my knowledge, no other method exists by which these locked-in accumulations may be eliminated from the body.

AN OVERVIEW OF THE PURIFICATION PROGRAM

$\mathcal{A}$ Word about the Program

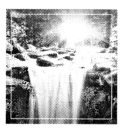

PART TWO, CHAPTER ONE

$\mathcal{A}$ WORD ABOUT THE PROGRAM

THE EXACT REGIMEN for the Purification Program is based on practical experience gained from the research and development of the program and through various pilot projects during which the program was delivered to thousands of individuals.

The established program procedure includes regulations that must be maintained and strictly adhered to.

1. This is *not* a program one should attempt to do on one's own. The Purification Program is an action that should be supervised and monitored by persons qualified and experienced in its delivery.

2. This program can be strenuous and should not be undertaken by anyone who has a weak heart or who is anemic. It is therefore absolutely essential that before participating in the Purification Program, one must first have a written medical authorization from an informed, licensed medical practitioner. If any signs of weak heart or anemia should appear while on the program, the person is taken off the program and directed to a medical practitioner.

People wishing to do the program who have a known heart condition, high blood pressure or anemia, or even those with certain kidney conditions, would require a program of a much lower gradient. If a person is unable to do the regular program for medical reasons, a medical doctor might recommend a less strenuous regimen of exercise and nutrition. However, this may require the medical doctor be personally involved in on-site supervision of the individual during participation in the program.

3. Women who are pregnant or breast-feeding should not do the program. It goes without saying, toxins that might have been lying dormant in the body could be released and some of these substances could be transmitted to the unborn child in utero or to an infant through the mother's milk.

Following the above helps to ensure the well-being of all participants.

EXERCISE AND SAUNA

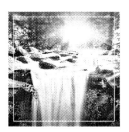

$\mathscr{E}$XERCISE AND $\mathscr{S}$AUNA

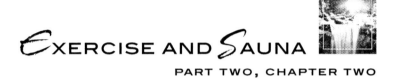

PART TWO, CHAPTER TWO

$\mathcal{T}$O FLUSH THE DRUGS and other chemical substances from the body, the Purification Program regimen begins with a combination of *exercise,* in the form of running, and *sauna.*

Running

The first action is running. The purpose of this is *not* to generate sweat, but to get the blood circulating and the system functioning so that impurities held in the system can be released and pumped out.

Running increases circulation throughout the whole body, thus:

1. It carries out cell waste more rapidly.
2. It causes the circulation to go deeper into the muscles and tissues so areas that have been stagnant can now get rid of the accumulation of biochemical deposits and, in the case of LSD, the "residual crystals" that have been stored.

Running is done daily once the person begins this program.

The intensity of running should be increased on a gradient. If you are so breathless that you can't talk to another while you are running, then you are straining too much. Reduce the intensity by running at a slower pace or for less time and then gradiently build the intensity as you progress through the program.

Sauna

The second action, following the running, is sweating in a sauna. The impurities can now be dispelled from the body and leave the system through the pores.

A sweat suit is *never* worn in the sauna, as this acts as insulation. One simply wears a swimsuit or some similar light apparel.

One should not get overheated in the sauna. If it gets too warm to comfortably tolerate the sauna heat, one would simply leave the sauna and take a cold shower. Then, once recovered, one would return to the sauna to again cause the body to sweat.

Of course, the objective of the Purification Program is to sweat out toxins, drugs and impurities from the system. The more time spent in the sauna, the faster progress one will make. However, one should not overdo it to the point of overheating and feeling faint or like keeling over! Instead, one should cool down in the shower when needed and then return to the sauna to continue sweating.

It is definitely *not* advisable to fall asleep in the sauna, as overheating could occur while one is asleep.

Running Time versus Sauna Time

On the Purification Program, five hours a day are spent on a combination of running and sweating.

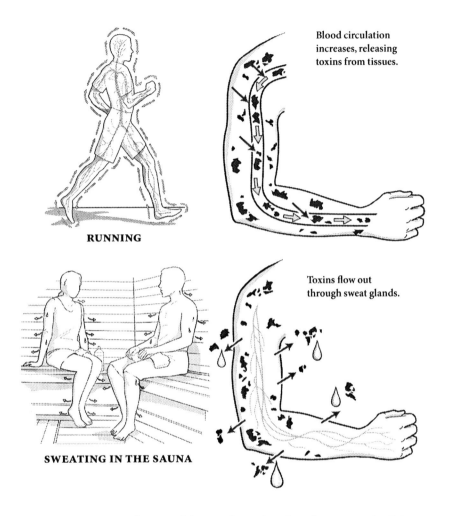

Blood circulation increases, releasing toxins from tissues.

RUNNING

Toxins flow out through sweat glands.

SWEATING IN THE SAUNA

It should be emphasized here that the five-hour period is *not* 50 percent running and 50 percent sauna. The program gives best results with a much lower percentage of time running and a much higher percentage in the sauna.

No arbitraries are set as to the exact time limits for each, but the bulk of the five-hour daily period of running and sauna sweat-out is best spent in the sauna after the circulation has been worked up by running.

One would not skimp on the running, however, as the most benefit is obtained from sweating when the circulation has been worked up so that the impurities are ready to be flushed out.

Running and sauna sweat-out must always be done with another person, as restimulation of past drugs, medicines, even anesthetics, can and often does occur as the toxins get sweated out. This can include the restimulation of a full-blown "trip" from LSD or the effects of other drugs one may have taken. It is a safeguard, therefore, to be accompanied by a partner or twin.

Liquids

While on this program, it is important to drink plenty of water. This greatly assists in flushing out and cleansing the system. Additionally, because of the amount of sweating one does in the sauna, the body's fluids must be replenished.

A sufficient intake of water is therefore quite vital when doing the program. This has a side effect, however, of washing a lot of minerals out of the system and perhaps vitamins as well. Thus the necessity of the intake of minerals and vitamins during the program.

One should *never* become dehydrated while on the program. To prevent this from occurring, the participant must drink plenty of water throughout the day, quite in addition to adequate and continuous intake while in the sauna.

Salt and Potassium

Salt (sodium chloride) is not mandatory for every individual on the program. It is only necessary as a treatment if the symptoms of salt depletion (heat exhaustion) are in evidence. Such symptoms include clammy skin, tiredness, weakness, headache, cramps, nausea, dizziness, vomiting or fainting.

As potassium is also lost in sweating, some of the above symptoms can stem from potassium depletion. If salt intake does not handle the above symptoms, one would switch to potassium gluconate tablets.

As an additional note, Bioplasma, also known as cell salts, may be used instead of salt tablets. As Bioplasma dissolves under the tongue, it is an alternative for those who have difficulty digesting salt in tablet form. Low-sodium "salt substitute" may also be used in place of potassium, as it is mainly potassium.

Lack of Sweating

If perspiration ceases while in the sauna, it needs to be addressed immediately. The most likely cause is lack of sufficient water intake. The handling is to get the body rehydrated by drinking sufficient water. This would occur with the person outside the sauna so that the body doesn't immediately sweat out the water taken in. If the person has become dehydrated to the point sweating has ceased to occur, it can take some time to rehydrate, since consumed water still has to be absorbed into the body. Drinking massive quantities of water all at once will not rectify the matter and is not advised. Rather, the correct thing to do is drink frequent small amounts of water until the symptoms of dehydration subside.

If the body suddenly stops sweating and the skin becomes hot and dry, this is the first sign of a heatstroke. This is the body clamping down and causing a resistance to expelling.

Should this occur, the person must immediately leave the sauna and cool off with a cold or cool shower or sponging, or start with a lukewarm shower and gradually make it cooler. Fluids, salt or potassium or Bioplasma would also be taken.

Everyone doing the program must be instructed on the above steps before they begin.

In summary, the three important points that must be in on a Purification Program are these:

1. Profuse sweating must occur.
2. A person's liquid intake must be large enough to compensate for the liquid lost through sweating.
3. Minerals and vitamins must be taken in sufficient quantities to replace those washed out of the system through sweating.

$\mathcal{D}$RUGS AND NUTRITIONAL DEFICIENCIES

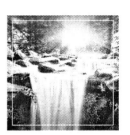

DRUGS AND NUTRITIONAL DEFICIENCIES

PART TWO, CHAPTER THREE

*M*ANY PEOPLE PROBABLY turn to drugs because they feel terrible as a result of unknown dietary deficiencies. This situation progressively worsens, as the drugs themselves cause wholesale vitamin and mineral deficiencies. Recovery from drugs, then, requires a full repair of dietary deficiencies.

Having been an early discoverer and instigator of vitamin therapy, I know whereof I speak on the subject of nutritional deficiencies. My work covering vitamins and deficiencies, stimulants and depressants and the field of biochemistry goes back to the spring of 1950 and earlier. Studies made in those fields were highly contributive to evolving the Purification Program.

Drugs and Toxins Equal Vitamin Burn-up

Toxins and drugs create vitamin and mineral deficiencies in the body. For example, a vitamin C deficiency, a B_1 deficiency, a B complex deficiency and a niacin deficiency are brought about by drugs. There may be other deficiencies caused by drugs that we are not aware of at this time, but that list is certain.

Also, alcohol, for example, depends for its effects upon a person being able to burn up B_1. When all of the B_1 in the system is burned up, the person goes into delirium tremens (D.T.'s) and nightmares.

In the case of other toxic substances, the probability exists that other vitamins are burned up. What we seem to have hit upon here is that LSD and other street drugs burn up not only B_1 and B complex, but also create a deficiency of niacin (one of the B complex vitamins) in the body and that the drugs possibly depend on niacin for their effect.

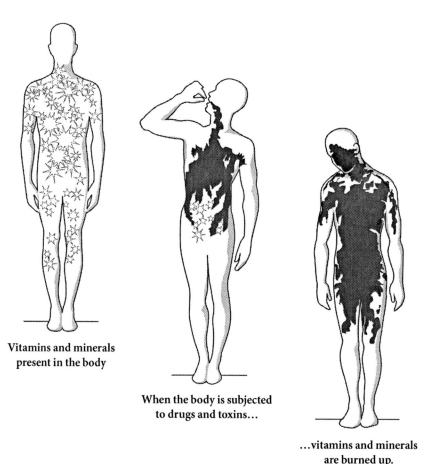

Vitamins and minerals
present in the body

When the body is subjected
to drugs and toxins...

...vitamins and minerals
are burned up.

In light of the discovery that toxic and drug residuals can remain in the body for years, it can be assumed that these residuals, to the degree that they are still present, might have the same and continuing effect on the body's vitamin and mineral reserves.

Deficiencies and Illness

Any vital substances on which body support depends, when too reduced or omitted from consumption, can be depended upon to result in a nonoptimum physical condition. When such an omission is very obvious, it becomes a "disease." When it is less obvious or even undetected, it becomes a "not feeling good."

A distinct possibility exists that, after mental and spiritual factors, the largest contributive factor in aging is the composite of cumulative deficiencies. Predisposition to other types of illness is, in many instances, occasioned by these deficiencies, even when the precipitation is viral or bacterial. Prolonged illness is guaranteed when deficiencies remain present and unremedied.

Thus a factor in the development of the Purification Program was to handle any such deficiencies with sufficient daily quantities of vitamins and minerals in addition to whatever was supplied through regular meals.

Creating Artificial Deficiencies

A vitamin or mineral does not work alone. It must combine with other elements to do its work. Lacking needed elements in one area, the body will rob bones, muscles and tissue to obtain the missing elements. Artificial deficiencies can be so created.

In fact, one can actually create a deficiency in vitamin C by administering B and calcium. All one has to do is pump those things into a person in very, very heavy dosages and they will develop the characteristics of C deficiency. Their teeth begin to hurt. Then when you give them C, the manifestations go away. The principle here is that by giving one or two vitamins in excess amount, you can create a nutritional deficiency of another vitamin that isn't being given or isn't being given in enough quantity.

The reason for this is that a vitamin makes certain changes in the body and these changes, to occur fully, also require the additional vitamin. But if that additional vitamin isn't present, the manifestation of being in deficiency is created.

When large dosages of certain vitamins, minerals or foodstuffs are given, an artificial deficiency can apparently be created in others not given. Increases in some elements, just by the fact of the increase, increases demand for others. When intake of some elements is markedly increased, balance must be maintained by proportionately increasing others. Thus vitamin rations on the Purification Program have to be taken in proportion to one another.

Minerals: Key to Glandular Interaction

Between 1945 and 1973, I studied the endocrine system. From this study, it seemed apparent that minerals and trace minerals operating in the bloodstream and circulated by other body fluids were a key to glandular interactions.

As various drugs upset the whole endocrine system of the body, administering vitamins and sweat-out and such actions create a mineral demand in the body. An imbalance of nutritional substances can also result in artificial *mineral* deficiencies. Therefore certain mineral dosages are given along with the rest of the program.

When one knows about nutrition and the elements of the program, it is obvious that, in the face of an unhandled mineral deficiency, the effectiveness of the procedure will suffer.

A Word about Diets

It should be noted that when we speak of *nutrition,* we are not talking only about vitamins and minerals; we are talking about food as well. All are vital to proper nutrition and the effectiveness of this program.

However, we are also not talking about "diet" in the common, overused sense of the word. There are *no* "diets" required on the Purification Program. Participants simply eat what they normally eat, supplemented with plenty of vegetables that have not been overcooked and with the needed dosages of vitamins and minerals. Vegetables contain a lot of minerals and fiber as well as some vitamins necessary to recovery.

There is no thought here of putting a person on any kind of special diet at all. There are no restrictions on what one may eat while on the program. We are not preaching against toxic foods or campaigning against diet abuses or junk foods or anything of that sort.

We are only trying to handle the *accumulation* of impurities built up in the body. If one wanted to defend one's body against all future impurities, then that is another program and not part of this one.

To put participants on an unaccustomed diet would introduce a sudden change in the midst of other changes they will experience on the program. A change of diet might be one too many changes and would be an additive that could interfere with and affect the efficacy of the program.

$\mathcal{N}$IACIN, THE "EDUCATED" VITAMIN

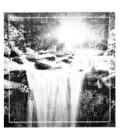

$\mathcal{N}$IACIN, THE "EDUCATED" VITAMIN

$\mathcal{N}$IACIN, AS ONE of the B complex vitamins, is essential to nutrition. It is so vital to the effectiveness of the Purification Program that it requires some extensive mention here. The biochemical reactions of niacin are my own discovery, made in the course of research spanning three decades.

Niacin can produce some startling and, in the end, very beneficial results when taken properly as part of the program (along with the other necessary vitamins and minerals in sufficient and proportionate quantities). But its effects can be quite dramatic and so one should have a good understanding of what niacin is and does before starting the Purification Program.

In particular, niacin appears to break up and unleash LSD from the tissues and cells. It can rapidly release LSD crystals into the system and send a person on a new "trip." (One fellow who had done the earlier Sweat Program for a period of months and who believed he had no more LSD in his system took 100 milligrams of niacin and promptly turned on a full-blown LSD "trip"!)

Niacin has the same effect on residues of marijuana and other drugs, along with various toxic substances. Hence this vitamin is an integral component to the Purification Program. Running and sweating must be done in conjunction with taking niacin to ensure the toxic substances released by niacin do get flushed from the body.

Niacin and Radiation

Among the most startling manifestations brought about by niacin is that it can turn on (cause to appear or activate) a past "sunburn." Remarkably, a red flush appears on a person's body, revealing the unmistakable outline of the bathing suit they were wearing when they were originally sunburned.

I first encountered this phenomenon in experiments I conducted in the 1950s. Strangely, at the time, both British and American pharmacopeias (books describing drugs and their uses) advertised that this substance, niacin, turned on a flush and inferred it was somehow toxic in high doses.

However, I discovered that if niacin was continued, in what the pharmacopeia would term "overdose," eventually one got no more flushes from it. Specifically the sunburnlike flushes would eventually disappear at a dosage of 200 milligrams, then at 500 milligrams they would recur but with less intensity. One might then get a small reaction for several days at 1,000 milligrams, after which one might administer 2,000 milligrams and find no more effects. The person would feel fine, the "sunburn" gone, and he would experience no more flush from the niacin.

But if niacin were toxic, how was it that the more one "overdosed" it, the sooner one no longer experienced the sunburnlike flushes from it?

The writers of the pharmacopeia or the biochemist may continue to think that niacin turns on a flush and that it will always turn on a flush in "overdoses." But the interesting part of it is the fact there comes a point when it *doesn't* turn on a flush. This doesn't happen by conditioning of the body; that is not what occurs.

Niacin will often cause a very hot flush and prickly, itchy skin, which can last up to an hour or longer. It may also bring on chills or make one feel tired. It appears that niacin *runs out* (releases and eliminates) something. In the case of the pattern of a bathing suit showing up, it is running out a sunburn, really a radiation burn. It also turns on nausea, skin irritation, hives and colitis, all of which are symptoms of radiation sickness.

Niacin, then, apparently has a catalytic effect on running out radiation exposure. So the Purification Program is not only for drugs: the quantities of niacin taken in combination with the heat of the sauna appear also to run out a certain amount of the accumulated radiation in people.

Running through Past Deficiencies

In theory, niacin apparently does not do anything by itself. It is simply interacting with niacin deficiencies that already exist in the cellular structure. For example, it does not turn on allergies; it appears to run out allergies. Evidently anything niacin does is the result of running out and running through past deficiencies.

The manifestations niacin produces can be quite amazing. Some of the somatics (physical pains or sensations) and manifestations have already been mentioned: LSD "trips," sunburns and the symptoms of radiation exposure. A person may also turn on flu symptoms, gastroenteritis, aching bones, upset stomach or even a fearful or terrified condition. In fact, there seems to be no limit to the variety of phenomena that may occur with niacin. If it is there to be run out by niacin, it apparently will do so with niacin.

The two vital facts proven by observation are these:

1. When the niacin was carried on until these things discharged, they did then vanish—as they *will* do.

   It is a matter of record that a reaction turned on by niacin will turn off where administration of niacin is continued.

2. When the niacin dosage was increased and the whole lot of the rest of the vitamins being taken was also increased proportionately, the niacin itself, taken in large amounts, did not create a vitamin deficiency.

On the program, therefore, the progressive increase of the niacin dosages determines the proportionate increase of the other vitamins and minerals. And in fact, it is niacin that monitors completion of the program, for when one no longer feels the effects of past drugs and toxins, one has achieved the product of the program itself.

Niacin's biochemical reaction was a pivotal discovery, one that made an incalculable contribution to the successful results of the Purification Program.

OIL: Trading Bad Fat for Good Fat

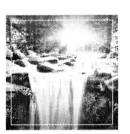

OIL: TRADING BAD FAT FOR GOOD FAT

PART TWO, CHAPTER FIVE

*A*S STATED PREVIOUSLY, toxic substances seem to lock up mainly, but not exclusively, in the fat tissues of the body. The goal, then, is to purge those substances from the fat tissues.

The theory at work on the Purification Program is that one could replace the fat tissues that hold these accumulations with fat that is free of such residues. The premise being, to get rid of something that is unwanted, one would have to give the body something as a substitute. So if a person takes some fat in the form of oil, the body might possibly exchange the bad fat in the body for the good oil. That is the basic theory.

I am indebted for material on this subject to a physician in Portugal who, in the course of my research, told me that doctors performing autopsies had found all sorts of gristly, used-up fat stored in unlikely places in people's bodies. In other words, a body can accumulate a lot of unusable fat.

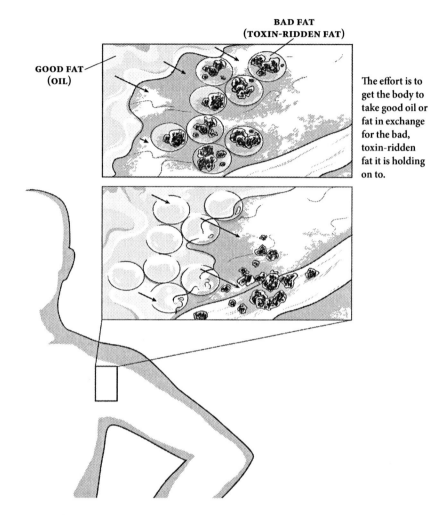

GOOD FAT
(OIL)

BAD FAT
(TOXIN-RIDDEN FAT)

The effort is to get the body to take good oil or fat in exchange for the bad, toxin-ridden fat it is holding on to.

The body will obviously hold on to a lot of fat and won't let go of it. The effort is to get the body to take good oil or fat in exchange for the bad, toxin-ridden fat it is holding on to.

All people, be they fat or thin, have some fatty tissue. Some, of course, have more fat stored in their bodies than others. On this program we simply want to get rid of the fat that contains the toxic substances; we are not even trying to make people lose weight. (Worth mentioning here is also the fact, particularly in regard to thin people, that while toxic substances lock up *mainly* in fat tissue, it does not mean that the person cannot have drug deposits inside other cells in the body.)

To promote the successful exchange of good fat for toxin-ridden fat, the correct oils must be taken as part of the Purification Program. These have been researched and include specific oils that contain essential fatty acids. *Fatty acids* are naturally occurring organic compounds that, according to nutritional researchers, are the key building blocks of all fats and oils, both in our foods and in our bodies. These compounds are vital to the construction and maintenance of all healthy cells. The essential fatty acids are called *essential* because they are fatty acids the body cannot make and must therefore acquire from food.

Along with the oil, a nutritional supplement called lecithin is also taken on the Purification Program. Lecithin, which comes in granulated form, appears to break up fat into tiny particles that can pass readily through the system.

If one wants to clean up the fat tissue in the body, one had better give the body some fat to make up for the fat tissues the body is now, on the Purification Program, releasing or changing.

The Importance of Calcium and Magnesium

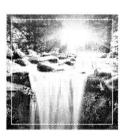

THE IMPORTANCE OF CALCIUM AND MAGNESIUM

PART TWO, CHAPTER SIX

ALTHOUGH BOTH CALCIUM and magnesium are usually included in the type of multimineral tablet which would be used on the Purification Program, additional dosages of these are an integral part of the program because of their particular effectiveness in helping to handle the effects of drugs.

Calcium: A Basic Building Block

Calcium is a must where any healing or exchange process is involved, as it is a basic building block of the body.

More important, calcium affects the nervous system.

I do not know the total relationship between calcium and toxic substances (and neither does anyone else), but it actually exists.

The rationale back of this is that a calcium deficiency sets up a person for spasms. Nerve spasms occur in the absence of calcium; muscular spasms are caused by lack of calcium. People who think they are in a state of high tension or something of the sort may simply have a calcium deficiency.

65

Calcium and Magnesium in Tandem

Magnesium is a mineral that has proven necessary to keep the nerves smoothed out. Magnesium, like calcium, is helpful in preventing sore muscles and so both are beneficial on the Purification Program.

However, in pairing these two minerals, yet another obstacle has to be overcome. Calcium must have an acidic base to operate in, while magnesium is an alkaline.

If the system is too alkaline, calcium will not release the positive ion that makes it possible for it to operate in the cellular structure and go through the vein walls, the intestinal walls and so forth. In other words, in an alkaline system calcium is ineffective and inactive.

Therefore I discovered the means of getting calcium and magnesium into solution in the body so that the results of both could be achieved. The breakthrough was to add vinegar, which creates the acidic base. With calcium, magnesium and vinegar in water, in exact ratio one to the other, the full benefits are achieved.

The result is a solution named the "Cal-Mag Formula." In addition to preventing sore muscles, Cal-Mag was found to have the added benefit of balancing certain vitamins on the Purification Program.

"FLASHBACKS," EMOTIONAL REACTIONS AND OTHER MANIFESTATIONS

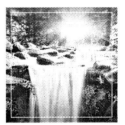

"_F_LASHBACKS," EMOTIONAL REACTIONS AND OTHER MANIFESTATIONS

PART TWO, CHAPTER SEVEN

_A_ N UNDERSTANDING OF the Purification Program would not be complete without a further discussion of the various manifestations that occur on the program. These can vary widely from person to person. Anything from an insect bite to a full-blown restimulation of an LSD "trip" may occur. When they do, they simply run their course and vanish as one continues through the daily regimen.

Program reports and medical case histories abound with statements from program participants wherein individuals identified the reactions they were going through with past on-the-job or other life experiences. These include, for example, reports of toxic exposure to vinyl paints, insecticides, paint thinner, a wide variety of industrial chemicals, preservatives, plant sprays and the like. Some have experienced sensations that they recognize or identify with previous X-ray treatments, dental procedures, anesthetics such as Novocain, or others from various operations, as well as any of the sensations that accompany various physical ills or injuries for which some type of medicine or drug was used.

Of course, also mentioned in no small measure are experiences with street drugs, or what are now termed in some quarters "recreational" drugs. Included in this category are marijuana, cocaine, heroin, hashish, LSD and so on. If there are drug residues to be flushed out, it is not uncommon for individuals to experience a restimulation of the exact effects of the drug or medicine from when they first took it.

Thus one might expect to encounter manifestations related to medical or pharmaceutical chemicals, over-the-counter medicines, industrial or household chemicals or hard street drugs. This phenomenon apparently can extend to any nutritional deficiency, or illness as a result of such deficiency, which has been caused by the ingestion or absorption of any of these chemical substances.

"Trips"

If a person is experiencing "trips" during the program, he should take extra vitamin B complex and vitamin C in correct ratio to other vitamins. These aid the body, especially the liver, in getting rid of the drugs in the system. It should be mentioned that the vitamins and minerals taken as part of the program are generally sufficient for the body to handle the residual drugs that are dislodged.

Aches, Pains, Somatics

Old injuries or old somatics may turn on, flare up for a brief period of time and then vanish. These may be sharply defined and easily recognized by the individual as related to some former experience. Or they may simply be vague feelings of discomfort that are not identified as relating to any one specific illness, injury or accident. These may range from headaches to muscular spasms, muscular aches, swellings, skin rashes, hives, bronchial symptoms or any number of other pains or somatics.

Sensations

Participants have also reported the following sensations while sweating out residuals in the sauna: light, "cloudy" feelings in the head, floating sensations, dizziness, feelings of being "spaced out" or "hung over" or numbness in the mouth around the gums and in some instances in the limbs or extremities.

They have further described any and all of the sensations associated with street drugs. Periods of intoxication (drunkenness) have reactivated briefly for some individuals while in the sauna and then dissipated and vanished.

Smells and Tastes

Very often a person will re-experience the smell or taste of some particular substance. Some of those described by program participants are an etherlike smell, the smell of marijuana, a metallic taste, the taste of Novocain, "a bitter taste," a "medicinelike" taste, a "chemicallike" taste, to name just a few.

These can also appear as unusual body odors emitted during periods of sweating in the sauna. One example is a participant who had worked for some time as a lifeguard at a swimming pool containing chlorinated water. For a certain period on the program, he exuded sweat with such a strong and overpowering smell of chlorine that others had to temporarily leave the sauna!

Emotions

Emotions that have been shut off or suppressed may also start to reappear. The person may go through emotional reactions connected with past biochemical experiences that dissipate over the course of the program. Individuals may also go through a period of dullness or stupidity and, as they come through it, become more aware. They may find they can then do actions more easily and consequences may start to take on a new meaning for them. Additionally, their memory can return.

Differences and Changes in Intensity

From reports based on direct observation, apparently what can happen in some cases (not all) is that the residuals of several past drugs and other chemicals (sometimes every drug or medicine the person has taken) can restimulate simultaneously and turn on heavily in the first week or ten days of the program at lower dosages of niacin. Others will experience these effects in a more graduated sequence, one following the other.

It doesn't always happen in an orderly fashion and in some instances it can be more severe than in others. But as a person sweats out the drug residuals and goes through any accompanying manifestations, the effects tend to become lighter and eventually there will be no effects, even when taking higher amounts of niacin.

A given manifestation may turn on, may or may not intensify, and then vanish wholly or partly in any one day. Then it may turn on again the following day but less intensely. If one increases the vitamin and mineral dosage at this time, the manifestation is likely to turn on again, but it will be milder. These manifestations don't become more and more severe, day by day; they become less and less so, day by day, providing the Purification Program is continued properly.

When the vitamins, minerals and other program actions no longer turn the manifestation on at all, it is gone. Evidence suggests that no amount of vitamin and mineral dosage above a certain final level for that individual will turn the manifestation on again.

Correct Gradient Is the Key

One of the keys to a successful Purification Program is to take the vitamins and mineral dosages in a proper gradient. Dosages that are too high too soon can turn a manifestation on awfully hard.

Where the person was on a sensible and well-kept schedule, with correct nutrient dosages and all other parts of the program followed, these manifestations deintensify and disappear without hanging up and without undue discomfort for the person. In other words, an individual may experience the effects caused by any nutritional deficiencies as well as the restimulative effects of toxic substances as they become active and discharge, but the person comes through these periods satisfactorily on a standard program.

Importance of a Proper Schedule

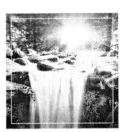

$\mathcal{I}$MPORTANCE OF A PROPER SCHEDULE

$\mathcal{I}$T IS IMPORTANT that a person participating in the Purification Program maintain a properly ordered schedule. This means once one has started on the program, one must stick to it sensibly and not skip days or do any part of it in a random fashion. To do otherwise may prevent a person from progressing smoothly through to successful completion of the program.

Optimum Daily Time on the Program

One's schedule must allow for the full time prescribed for the Purification Program. From the many cases interviewed and from those who have supervised the program, the optimum daily time on the program is five hours, the bulk of which is spent in the sauna.

Not everyone has gone immediately on to a full five-hour period right from the start. Among the many surveyed were those who required a few days to work up to five hours daily, but once they reached that schedule, it proved to be the optimum daily time period for them.

It has been found that some enthusiastic participants have overdone it at the start. This was remedied by having them work up gradually to running twenty to thirty minutes without strain, while increasing the sauna time gradually to the full prescribed period.

Doing the Program on Less Than Five Hours Daily

In cases where persons have limited time due to an inflexible schedule, a shorter schedule can be arranged, as it would be inappropriate to deny them the program. But it is necessary to ensure that each person can, and does, make progress on the shorter daily schedule. If one does not, one would need to be put on to a longer regimen.

Shorter schedules range from four hours down to the absolute minimum of two and one-half hours daily, always with a higher percentage of time spent in the sauna than running—approximately 20–30 minutes of running and the remaining time in the sauna.

Some who start at two and one-half hours daily later request to move up to the five-hour period. In some cases persons on the shorter schedule experienced heavy restimulation of drugs, which did not fully run its course on the shorter period, but when switched to the five-hour period did remarkably better.

Time Factors for a Person with Extensive Drug History

All research and survey data thus far indicate that the extent of drug history is definitely a factor in determining how much daily time an individual would spend on the program.

Beyond any doubt, the surveys show that those with heavy or even mediumly heavy drug histories benefited most from the five-hour daily schedule. This can apply to persons with heavy medical-drug histories as well as to those who have taken heavy street drugs.

Persons with heavy drug histories have reported that if something turned on while in the sauna, they made it a point to stick carefully to the sauna time (taking short breaks as necessary for water, salt or potassium or to cool off) until the manifestation blew (went away) after which they came out feeling good and refreshed. These same persons reported that if they shortcut the sauna time because something uncomfortable had turned on, they came out feeling bad or dull and it would then take longer for the manifestation to run its course.

Even some people with very light drug histories reported feeling calmer and more upbeat after a period in the sauna that was long enough to permit them to get through any restimulation or discomfort that had turned on.

There is everything to be said for putting individuals on a schedule that will permit them to handle these factors so that they are able to get full return from the program.

Program Irregularities

Probably the biggest single factor found to prevent a person from progressing smoothly through to successful completion of the program was *irregularity* of schedule, nutrition and any other part of the regimen.

When any one part was done erratically, it threw the other parts out.

According to surveys, when people who had otherwise been doing well began skipping a day here or there, skimping or cutting down on the daily regimen, it usually resulted in some degree of discomfort.

The handling was to get the person back on to a proper and predictable daily regimen and maintain it through to completion of the program.

During the period on the Purification Program, one should follow normal and generally accepted rules for good health and be in the best possible shape to help attain the lasting spiritual benefits that are available on the program. This is, of course, the sole and ultimate objective of the Purification Program.

Sleep

By far the most common schedule deviation found, from those reporting any difficulties on the program, was lack of sufficient sleep.

The need for adequate sleep cannot be overemphasized.

As borne out in participant reports, the Purification Program can be strenuous. A person observably needs enough sleep and rest to cope with the changes taking place in his body and to assist the rebuilding of tissues or cellular repair.

Eight hours of sleep is considered the usual daily requirement. Some persons may need more than this, but getting less than the regular amount of sleep one usually requires is not advised. People function best when they are sufficiently rested.

One obviously cannot expect to make the gains possible on the Purification Program unless this point is observed.

Length of Program

Taking into account all of the above, at five hours a day one should be able to get through the whole program in three to four weeks, although some will take more and some will take less. But regardless of length, the Purification Program provides all participants the process by which they can take a vital step toward a toxin-free, drug-free life.

COMPLETING THE PURIFICATION PROGRAM

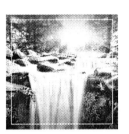

COMPLETING THE PURIFICATION PROGRAM

THE OBJECTIVE OF the Purification Program is very simply to clean out and purify one's system of all the accumulated impurities, such as drugs and other toxic substances—e.g., food preservatives, insecticides, pesticides, etc. For someone who has taken LSD, this includes getting rid of any residual crystals from the body.

One is complete with the program when one is free of the restimulative presence of residuals from past chemicals, drugs and toxins. One will no longer feel the effects of these impurities going into restimulation and usually will report a marked resurgence of vitality and an overall sense of well-being. These indicators, which are present when the action has been fully and correctly completed, are known as the END PHENOMENA.

Obviously if a person is still feeling the effects of past drugs or chemicals going into restimulation, the program cannot be considered complete and must be continued until all these manifestations have turned off completely.

The product of the Purification Program is a purified body, free from accumulated impurities, drugs and other toxins that could prevent one's mental and spiritual advance.

~

$\mathcal{A}$ New Life
THROUGH PURIFICATION

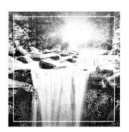

A New Life THROUGH PURIFICATION

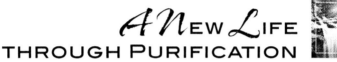

*W*ITH THE PURIFICATION PROGRAM we now have the means to get rapid recovery from the effects of the accumulation of environmental chemical poisons as well as medical and street drugs.

With the inclusion of a precise regimen of vitamins, minerals and oils, we are able to work toward restoring the biochemical balance of the body and make it possible for the body to reconstruct itself from the damage done by drugs and other biochemical substances.

In so doing we are able to bring individuals up to the level where they are now on the path toward mental and spiritual gain.

From this step alone they will see some sparkling results.

The Purification Program gives an individual the chance to experience a surge of vitality and renewed sense of well-being.

It is offered as an invitation to start living!

DRUGS AND SOCIETY

CLEAR BODY, CLEAR MIND

MORE ON DRUGS AND THEIR EFFECTS

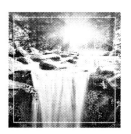

$\mathcal{M}$ORE ON $\mathcal{D}$RUGS AND THEIR EFFECTS

DRUGS AND SOCIETY

*I*F ONE IS TO fully address the agonizing effects of drugs—and there is too much at stake in terms of human life *not* to make an attempt to do so—it is necessary to gain a greater understanding of what drugs really do to the body and mind.

"If You Are Numb, Nothing Can Hurt You"

Drug users, from observation, are apparently sitting on the fallacy that "If you are numb, nothing can hurt you." Drugs, then, are probably a defense against the travails of everyday living. They do block off pain and other unwanted sensations. But there is a whole sector of *desirable* sensations and drugs block off *all* sensations.

Sexually it is common for someone on drugs to be very stimulated at first. This is the "procreate before death" impulse. In other words, as drugs are poisons, the body instinctively perceives a threat to its survival and so strives to reproduce. But after the original sexual "kicks," the stimulation of sexual sensation becomes harder and harder to achieve. The effort to achieve becomes obsessive while the actual act is less and less satisfying. In spite of propaganda to the contrary, even sexual sensation is blocked off with drugs and this is true even after drugs have apparently heightened it one or two times. After that it is dead, dead, dead.

Emotion, Perception and Somatic Shut-off

Those who have been long and habitually on drugs, medicine or alcohol sometimes suffer from emotional, perception or somatic (physical pains or sensations) shut-offs. They appear anesthetized (unfeeling) and sometimes have "nothing troubling them," whereas they are, in reality, in a suppressed mental and physical condition and cannot stop taking drugs or drink or medicine.

These individuals took up drugs, alcohol or medicine as a cure for unwanted pain, sensation or feelings.

The only statement that can be made for drugs is that they give a short, quick oblivion from immediate agony and permit the handling of a person to effect repair. But even this is applicable only to persons who have no other system to handle their pain.

Dexterity, ability and alertness are the main things that prevent getting into painful situations and these all vanish with drugs. So drugs set individuals up to get into situations that are truly disastrous and they keep them that way.

One has a choice between being dead with drugs or being alive without them. Drugs rob life of the sensations and joys that are the only reasons for living anyhow.

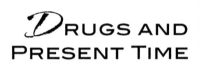Drugs and Present Time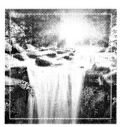

DRUGS AND PRESENT TIME

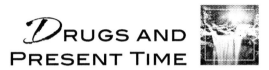

DRUGS AND SOCIETY

WHILE DRUG USERS consider drugs valuable to the degree they produce some "desirable effect," people on drugs are dangerous to others around them because drugs have unpredictable effects. Individuals under the influence of drugs have blank periods, unrealities and delusions that remove them from "present time."

Present time is a very important factor in mental and spiritual sanity and ability. Human beings can be stuck in literally thousands of different past moments. Their behavior and attitudes are influenced by such past incidents and experiences.

Drugs may drive a person out of an unbearable present time or out of consciousness altogether. Afterwards some people do not wholly return to present time. Thus right before your eyes the person, apparently in the same room as you are, doing the same things, is really only partially there and partially in some past event. He *seems* to be there, but really he isn't tracking fully with present time.

What is going on, to a rational observer, is *not* what is going on to this individual. He does not fully comprehend statements made by another, but tries to fit them into his composite reality. To fit them in, the individual has to alter them.

He may be *sure* he is helping you *repair* the floor when what you are doing actually is *cleaning* the floor. So his actions (which seem logical and correct to him) are actually hindering the operation in progress. Thus when he "helps you" mop the floor, he introduces chaos into the activity. Since in his mind he is *repairing* the floor, a request to "Give me the mop" gets reinterpreted as "Hand me the hammer." But the mop handle is larger than a hammer, so the bucket gets upset, with suds and water splashed all over the place.

That is a mild example—the kind of thing that doesn't make the headlines. But what of the accidents, the crimes, the despair that lead to all manner of tragedies that do make the headlines?

Because an individual can come up with an infinity of combinations, there is an infinity of types of reactions to drugs.

What is *constant,* however, is that the person who has used drugs is *not running in the same series of events* as others.

This difference can be slight, wherein the person makes occasional mistakes. Or the difference can be as serious as total insanity, where the events apparent to them are *completely* different than those apparent to everyone else. And there can be all gradients in between.

It isn't that these people don't know what's going on. It is that they perceive *something else* going on instead of the actual present time series of events that is happening.

This information can help one understand what may lie beneath the mistakes and erratic behavior of one's co-workers, friends and family members. The Purification Program offers such individuals the road out from the shadows of the past into present time.

DRUGS AND LEARNING

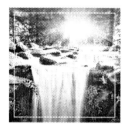

$\mathcal{D}$RUGS AND $\mathcal{L}$EARNING

DRUGS AND SOCIETY

IN VIEW OF ALL the effects brought about by drugs, one might easily deduce that drugs impede learning. But the statement is more than a simple deduction: it is empirical fact. Learning rate—the length of time it takes someone to learn something—has been proven to be slower in drug users than others. Actual tests show that the learning rate of a person who has been on drugs is much lower than that of a person who has not been on drugs.

Drugs, then, prevent a person from being educated. Weigh this against the fact that drug usage among students is not only tolerated in many schools and colleges, but some drugs are even *employed throughout the educational system*. One example of this is the use of prescribed psychiatric drugs as a means to handle what is termed "attention deficit."

Drug use may, indeed, be at the root of the widely publicized problems with current education. Teachers have been cited, in various articles in the press and other media, for failure or inability to teach. The problem may not rest with the teachers at all, but the drugs they have taken. Now, after decades of spreading and accelerating drug usage, a generation of students affected by drugs are now themselves teachers attempting to educate the next generation, which is *also* being influenced and affected by drugs.

Whatever the actual statistics may be on that score, it is certain that drugs are prevalent in schools. It is also certain that drugs impede learning and thus impede education.

Learning Rate and Criminality

The memory inspired by drugs often removes the drug user and former drug user from fear of consequences for any of their actions. One might think that the answer is discipline. But discipline is enforced learning. If attempts to simply teach an individual fail in the face of impeded learning, attempts to teach by discipline and justice actions—enforced learning—fail harder still. People who cannot learn and who are then subjected to forced learning by disciplinary action simply become criminals.

What good does it do a government to try to get police and justice actions into effect in a society that cannot learn? Governmental threats in a society that cannot learn are of no use. Society does not learn from such threats, therefore it wouldn't matter what measures the government took. A society that cannot learn, which is then subjected to attempted enforced learning, in the end becomes criminal.

A civilization that cannot be educated, that cannot learn, cannot last. This means *this* civilization will be ended unless something is done about it. The Purification Program holds hope for those affected by past drug use to gain the ability to learn.

$\mathcal{P}$AINKILLERS

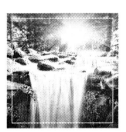

$\mathcal{P}$AINKILLERS

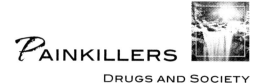

DRUGS AND SOCIETY

$\mathcal{D}$URING MY EARLY research on drugs, I made a breakthrough on the action of painkillers (such as aspirin, tranquilizers, hypnotics and soporifics).

At that time it had never been known in chemistry or medicine (and I am not sure that it is generally known today) exactly how or why these things worked. Such compositions are derived by accidental discoveries that "such and so depresses pain."

The effects of existing compounds are not uniform in result and often have very bad side effects.

As the reason they worked was unknown, very little advance has been made in biochemistry. If the reason they worked were known and accepted, possibly chemists could develop some actual compounds that would have minimal side effects.

Pain or discomfort of a psychosomatic nature comes from mental image pictures. These pictures of perceptions from the past can be restimulated and affect an individual physically.

By actual clinical test, the actions of aspirin and other pain depressants are these:

1. To inhibit the ability of the individual to create mental image pictures.
2. To impede the electrical conductivity of nerve channels.

With this, people are rendered stupid, blank, forgetful, delusive, irresponsible. They get into a "wooden" sort of state, unfeeling, insensitive, unable and definitely not trustworthy—a menace to their fellows, actually.

When the drugs wear off or start to wear off, the ability to create mental image pictures starts to return and *turns on* physical pains and sensations *much harder*. One of the answers a person has for this is *more* drugs. To say nothing of heroin, there are aspirin addicts. The compulsion stems from a desire to get rid of the somatics and unwanted sensations again. There is also some evidence of dramatization of the pictures turned on from earlier drug taking. The person gets more and more wooden, requiring more and more quantity and more frequent use of the drug.

To paraphrase an old adage, we used to have iron men and wooden ships. We now have a drug society and wooden citizens.

If one were working on this biochemically, the least harmful pain depressant would be one that inhibited the creation of mental image pictures with minimal resulting "woodenness" or stupidity and which was body-soluble so that it passed rapidly out of the nerves and system. There are no such biochemical preparations at this time.

The medical aspect is an understandable wish to handle pain. Doctors should press for better drugs to do this that do not have such lamentable side effects. Drug companies would be advised to do better research. The formula of least harmfulness is that given above.

SOLUTIONS FOR DRUG ADDICTION

CLEAR BODY, CLEAR MIND

$\mathcal{W}$ITHDRAWAL FROM ADDICTIVE DRUGS

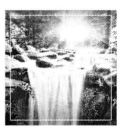

$\mathcal{W}$ITHDRAWAL FROM ADDICTIVE DRUGS

SOLUTIONS FOR DRUG ADDICTION

$\mathcal{T}$HE PURIFICATION PROGRAM is not administered to those currently addicted to drugs, though such persons need this program even more urgently, perhaps, than others. Thus a workable withdrawal program must precede the Purification Program for individuals who are addicted and cannot easily stop on their own.

These withdrawal procedures are part of the drug rehabilitation technology I developed earlier and which is in broad use by Narconon rehabilitation centers.

Withdrawal Symptoms

The most wretched part of coming off hard drugs is the associated withdrawal symptoms. These are the physical and mental reactions to no longer taking drugs. They are ghastly. No torturer ever set up anything worse. These reactions can be so severe that the addict becomes very afraid of them and so remains on drugs. Indeed, some individuals experience convulsions, and extreme withdrawal reactions can even include death.

It used to be that individuals on drugs had these options:

1. Stay on drugs and be trapped and suffering from there on out.
2. Try to come off drugs and be so agonizingly ill meanwhile that they couldn't tolerate it.

It was a "dead if you do, dead if you don't" sort of problem.

Medicine did not solve it adequately. Psychotherapy was impossible.

Handling Withdrawal

Fortunately, at least three approaches now exist for this problem.

1. Light objective processes (techniques that help individuals to look or place their attention outward from themselves). These processes, which I developed in the 1950s, have been put to effective use in helping to get through withdrawal with a minimum of pain.
2. Nutritional therapy. Instead of just telling individuals to break off drugs, with all that suffering and danger of failure, they are given heavy doses of vitamins and minerals, which have been found to be beneficial in assisting withdrawal.
3. Calcium and magnesium, taken in the Cal-Mag Formula.

The use of Cal-Mag, piloted in the early '70s to help ease withdrawal symptoms, is now long past the experimental stage. Cal-Mag has been used very effectively during withdrawal to help ease and counteract the convulsions, muscular spasms and severe nervous reactions experienced by an addict when coming off drugs. Effective in withdrawal from any drug, Cal-Mag has been reported as most radically, observably effective with methadone and heroin cases.

As calcium and magnesium are minerals, not drugs, one is not adding to the drug effects the person is already suffering. Rather, one is providing those minerals that are certain to be in deficiency in such cases and helping to provide some relief from the agonizing effects of such deficiencies.

Methadone, for example, attacks bone marrow and bones. Therefore one usually encounters a severe depletion of calcium in methadone users, characterized by severe pain in joints and bones, teeth problems, hair loss. Getting calcium into the system (in the acidic base in which it can operate) along with magnesium (for its effect on the nerves) helps to relieve these conditions. It has been reported that with use of Cal-Mag a person can be withdrawn from methadone anywhere from two weeks to three months faster than without its use. This may apply in withdrawal from other drugs as well.

Since drugs or alcohol rapidly burns up the vitamin B_1 in the system, taking a lot of B_1 daily when coming off drugs helps to avoid the convulsions that often attend this deficiency. The B_1 must, of course, be flanked with other increased vitamin dosages to maintain a proper balance of needed nutrients. Accordingly sufficient quantities of Cal-Mag and other minerals are also needed, both to prevent created mineral deficiencies and to work their wonders in easing and relieving the agonies accompanying withdrawal.

From one to three glasses of Cal-Mag a day, with or after meals, *replace any tranquilizer*. Cal-Mag does not produce the drugged effects of tranquilizers (which are quite deadly).

As withdrawal symptoms can be so terrible (and so lacking in success have the medical and psychiatric fields been in countering these reactions), the full data on the use of these vital minerals to counteract withdrawal symptoms should be broadly known.

Vitamins, Minerals and Oil

Vitamin and Mineral Tables

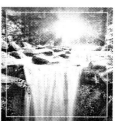

VITAMIN AND MINERAL TABLES

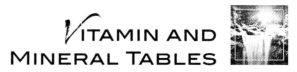

VITAMINS, MINERALS AND OIL

*T*HE TABLES ON the following pages provide the approximate gradient increases of vitamins and minerals taken as a person progresses through the Purification Program.

The recommended dosages in these tables, gathered through research, show the variations of individual tolerances encountered and the ranges of increase which have proven most effective in the majority of cases.

The figures on these tables designating points of increase (Stages 1, 2, 3, 4 and 5) do *not* refer to the first, second, third, fourth and fifth days of the program. They refer to approximate "stages" of vitamin and mineral increase in relation to the increased niacin.

Under Stage 1 on the Vitamin and Mineral Tables, the first figure given for each supplement shows the usual starting dosage for most individuals. The range of each vitamin and mineral in Stage 1 indicates how beginning dosages are increased depending upon the niacin reaction the person is experiencing. As the effects of the niacin diminish, the niacin is increased on a gradient. In this way, one would get an overlap of the old dosage having no effect and the new dosage being needed. Increasing the niacin dosage each time the effect of a dosage diminished (as opposed to having no effect) was found to speed up progress through the program considerably.

As an example, a person starts the program on 100 milligrams of niacin, plus beginning dosages of the other vitamins and minerals per the tables. He continues with these daily dosages until the effects of the niacin diminish. In his case, this occurs on, let us say, the third day. At that point, his niacin dosage is increased to 200 milligrams, with other vitamins and minerals increased proportionately. The person would carry on with those dosages until the niacin effects again lessen. Progressing in this way, by the seventh day of the program his vitamins and minerals may have been increased to the levels given in Stage 2 of the tables. After the ninth day, his vitamins and minerals may have increased all the way to Stage 3 of the tables. And he continues in this manner all the way to the dosage levels at Stage 5.

There is no rote formula to be followed in increasing the dosage of niacin and the other vitamins and minerals. In some cases, the niacin reaction may have been so strong that only a 100 milligram increase is indicated. Then, as the individual continues, the reactions may have lessened to the degree that a several hundred or even 500 milligram increase may be appropriate. Reactions can also vary widely one person to the next. Therefore it is a matter of those supervising the program increasing the dosages based on the participant's reaction to the niacin:

- Increasing the niacin dosage when the effects from the current dosage have diminished.
- Increasing the niacin dosage by an appropriate amount based on the individual's reaction and what he can tolerate.

Vitamin Table

This table shows proportionate vitamin increases at various stages of the program.

	STAGE 1	STAGE 2	STAGE 3	STAGE 4	STAGE 5
Niacin (mg)	100–400	500–1,400	1,500–2,400	2,500–3,400	3,500–5,000
Vitamin A (IU)	5,000–10,000	20,000	30,000	40,000	50,000
Vitamin D (IU)	400	800	1,200	1,600	2,000
Vitamin C (gm)	.25–1	2–3	3–4	4–5	5–6
Vitamin E (IU)	800	1,200	1,600	2,000	2,400
Vitamin B Complex	2 tablets	3 tablets	4 tablets	5 tablets	6 tablets
Vitamin B_1 (mg)	350–600	400–650	450–700	750–1,250	800–1,300

Mineral Table

The following table lays out the approximate mineral amounts found to give best results at the various stages of vitamin increase. The minerals listed are those generally found combined in multimineral tablets.

	STAGE 1	STAGE 2	STAGE 3	STAGE 4	STAGE 5
Calcium (mg)	500– 1,000	1,000– 1,500	1,500– 2,000	2,000– 2,500	2,500– 3,000
Magnesium (mg)	250– 500	500– 750	750– 1,000	1,000– 1,250	1,250– 1,500
Iron (mg)	18–36	36–54	54–72	72–90	90–108
Zinc (mg)	15–30	30–45	45–60	60–75	75–90
Manganese (mg)	4–8	8–12	12–16	16–20	20–24
Copper (mg)	2–4	4–6	6–8	8–10	10–12
Potassium (mg)	45– 90	90– 135	135– 180	180– 225	225– 270
Iodine (mg)	.225– .450	.450– .675	.675– .900	.900– 1.125	1.125– 1.350
Cal-Mag	1 to 1½ glasses	1 to 2 glasses	1 to 2 glasses	2 to 3 glasses	2 to 3 glasses

Final Stage of Niacin

Most persons on the Purification Program reach the niacin dosage of 5,000 milligrams, the final stage on the preceding Vitamin Table. When no further reaction occurs at this dosage and they have achieved the End Phenomena, they are complete.

However, a few individuals reach 5,000 milligrams but continue to experience a slight flush, day after day, with no other manifestations. If the person has done the program standardly and has achieved the End Phenomena, it has been found unnecessary to endlessly continue at 5,000 milligrams because of the slight flush.

Vitamins and Minerals after Completing the Program

A continuation of the vitamins, minerals, oil, vegetables and Cal-Mag is wise after completing the program. After taking heavy dosages of vitamins and minerals in the final stage of the program, to abruptly stop taking them could produce a letdown. Therefore the individual should come down from high dosages on a steep gradient to what would be normal recommended daily requirements. That, along with some moderate daily exercise, will also help the person maintain good health.

The research data offered here is not to be construed as a recommendation of medical treatment or medication. It is provided as a record of food supplements in the form of the nutritional vitamins and minerals which were used in the development of the Purification Program and which were found to be most effective in the greatest number of cases.

CALCIUM AND MAGNESIUM: THE CAL-MAG FORMULA

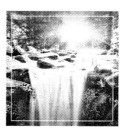

*C*ALCIUM AND MAGNESIUM: THE CAL-MAG FORMULA

VITAMINS, MINERALS AND OIL

*T*HE CAL-MAG FORMULA uses the following compounds: calcium gluconate and magnesium carbonate. Both of these come in white, powdery form. Each is a compound of different substances. In other words, calcium gluconate contains other substances besides calcium; it is not all pure calcium, but contains only a percentage of pure elemental calcium. Similarly magnesium carbonate contains other substances besides magnesium and includes only a percentage of pure elemental magnesium. By *elemental* is meant of chemical elements that are uncombined with other chemicals.

The following is the precise recipe for the Cal-Mag Formula.

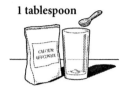

1. Put 1 level tablespoon of calcium gluconate in a normal-sized glass.

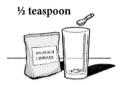

2. Add ½ level teaspoon of magnesium carbonate.

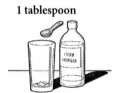

3. Add 1 tablespoon of cider vinegar (at least 5 percent acidity).

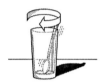

4. Stir it well.

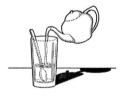

5. Add ½ glass of boiling water and stir until all the powder is dissolved and the liquid is clear. (If this doesn't occur, it could be a result of poor-grade or old magnesium carbonate.)

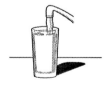

6. Fill the remainder of glass with lukewarm or cold water and cover. The solution will keep for up to two days.

Measures and Metric System Equivalents

For parts of the world that do not use the English system of weights and measures, the metric-system equivalents will clear up any possible question as to the proportions to be used in the formula.

One tablespoon per the English system of weights and measures = 15 milliliters (14.7 ml to be exact) per the metric system.

One teaspoon per the English system of weights and measures = 5.0 milliliters (4.9 ml to be exact) per the metric system.

These figures can be rounded off because the differences are so slight as to be negligible and, rounded, they remain in correct ratio.

Substituting these metric equivalents would give a Cal-Mag Formula as follows:

1. Put 15 ml calcium gluconate in a normal-sized glass.
2. Add 2.5 ml magnesium carbonate.
3. Add 15 ml of cider vinegar (at least 5 percent acidity).
4. Stir it well.
5. Add ½ glass (or about 120 ml) of boiling water and stir until all the powder is dissolved and the liquid is clear. (If this doesn't occur, it could be a result of poor-grade or old magnesium carbonate.)
6. Fill the remainder of glass with lukewarm or cold water and cover.

$\mathcal{O}$ILS

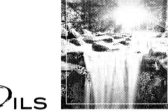

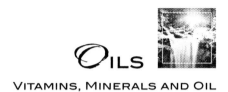

Oils

VITAMINS, MINERALS AND OIL

"ALL BLEND" IS the oil generally used on the Purification Program. It is a combination of different types of oils that contain essential fatty acids.

Essential Fatty Acids

The two basic types of essential fatty acids are omega-3 and omega-6.

Some oils that contain omega-3 are flax and walnut. Sources for omega-6 include oils such as soy, safflower, peanut and olive. Both categories contain many oils, but those above have been found to be effective on the Purification Program. Others may be effective as well.

According to researchers, the optimum ratio of omega-3s to omega-6s in a person's diet ranges from 1:1 to 4:1. In other words, one to four parts omega-3 to one part omega-6. Therefore the blend of oils used on the Purification Program generally falls within this range.

If an individual is allergic to any particular oil, he would replace it with one he is not allergic to.

When mixing individual oils (and not using All Blend), one should:

1. Obtain cold-pressed and polyunsaturated oils that contain the correct essential fatty acids.
2. Combine two or more oils in the correct ratio.
3. Refrigerate the oil blend so it does not go rancid.

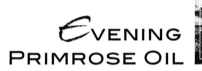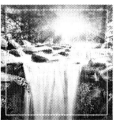

Evening Primrose Oil

*E*VENING PRIMROSE OIL

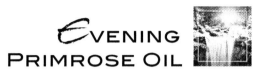

VITAMINS, MINERALS AND OIL

*E*VENING PRIMROSE OIL is another oil that has been found beneficial for some participants on the Purification Program.

Evening primrose oil is extracted from the crushed seeds of the evening primrose plant and is available in capsule form from many health-food stores. According to researchers, it purportedly handles various food allergies and seems to help break down dietary fat and fatty tissue.

It has been reported that some Purification participants evidence trouble metabolizing fat while on the program. Factors that may suggest an inability to metabolize fat range from the presence of gallstones to feeling nauseated, or sick to the stomach, after taking the oils.

Persons who have manifested difficulty metabolizing fat while on the program sometimes appeared to benefit when evening primrose oil was added to their daily regimen of oil and vitamins. Some of those apparently assisted were persons who previously had difficulties metabolizing fat (as indicated by a lack of weight loss when moderately dieting) and a few persons with heavy drug or alcohol histories (found on medical examination to have unhealthy livers) that inhibited their ability to metabolize fat. Evening primrose oil also seemed to assist some participants who had trouble metabolizing the All Blend oil.

Evening primrose oil is not taken by every participant, but does appear to be beneficial for some persons who may have difficulty metabolizing fat while on the Purification Program.

Purification Program Results

CLEAR BODY, CLEAR MIND

PROGRAM PARTICIPANT SUCCESSES

*S*INCE IT BEGAN in 1979, two major factors have contributed to the Purification Program's phenomenal success.

The first is the growing public awareness of the enormous quantity of drugs, toxins and chemicals in our world and their harmful effects on our lives.

The second factor is, of course, the program's *results*. The testimonials of those whose lives were radically improved come from all parts of the world and speak for themselves.

While no claim is made regarding what the program will specifically do for any one person, the following statements are representative of the results tens of thousands have achieved by completing the Purification Program.

DRUGS, ALCOHOL, MEDICINES AND TOXINS

Drugs and Alcohol

As a result of doing the Purification Program, I am much, much, MUCH more alert, aware and awake, with an abundance of energy with which to live life. Before participating in this program, I had no idea what the adverse effects of drugs had been upon me. I had taken various street drugs and my belief was that this was "behind" me. I was wrong. I was in fact carrying with me, every day of my life, the residual effects of these poisons.

Most notable was LSD. This is an insidious drug which affects one's perception of reality and ability to think. I once believed that this drug could take me to some new height of spiritual/mental awareness. Now, having done the Purification Program, it is very clear that the exact opposite was the case. To be rid of its effects is definitely a relief and my increased energy, productivity and zest for life is a testimony to this fact.

This program was a true lifesaver and it gave me a whole new and refreshing outlook on life. My thanks to L. Ron Hubbard for his work and brilliance in devising this fantastic program which helps people so greatly to achieve their full potential in living.

–F.S.

~

Before the Purification Program I was agitated all the time. I was just not being comfortable ever and I would get easily bugged by people. I didn't feel relaxed and I felt really tense. I would wake up in a bad mood or I'd just be in a bad mood for no reason.

While I was on the program, I would feel totally stoned, like I had just smoked pot. I knew I was running out marijuana, as I'd either be really lethargic or goofy. I ran out cocaine and would get really agitated and start talking a lot. I took LSD one time before and I felt this metallic, nasty taste in my mouth. I'm like, cool, get it out, get it out, I don't ever want it to come back!

Since I've finished, my perceptions are better; how I think about things is clearer; my eyesight is sharper and clearer; I'm happier. I'm not agitated.

I'm just being me and not feeling like a piece of wood, but feeling like a live person and being extroverted and enjoying life.

–K.K.

~

The Purification Program was exactly what I needed. For a long time I felt like I was walking around in a fog. I felt bad physically and was not sure why. By the second day I realized that it was all the drugs that were in my body for many, many years. After each day I felt brighter, more clear, calmer and more stable as a being. I handled not being able to study (something I had struggled with for years) and suddenly completed my course and read four books in a few days (I hadn't read a book for enjoyment in ten years). The best part is being able to see for what feels like the first time in a long time. This action absolutely changed me and gave me a new attitude on life.

–E.C.

~

I never truly realized what alcohol can do to not only your body, but to your mind. And the emotions and restimulation that occurred from the incidents attached to drinking. Incidents hang you up in the areas, leaving them susceptible to restimulation that really knocked me around in life and in the sauna! Now I really feel sharp again. Much more calm.

I really feel as though a big weight has been lifted off my mind, and my body. I wake up feeling good. I forgot this was how you're supposed to feel!

–J.X.

~

The Purification Program saved my life! I was totally unaware of the bad effects of drugs and toxins on my physical and mental well-being. I felt that I'd "ruined" my full potential because I'd taken drugs when I was young, that I'd never make up the time I lost and the reserves I'd wasted being addicted to drugs.

In addition to all the incredible gains I've gotten from the Purification Program, that sense of being limited by past mistakes is totally gone and my perception of my true potential is that it is limitless.

–M.B.

~

I was drinking a lot. I had just graduated from college and still was in my party mode. I was sort of confused in my life and having trouble making decisions clearly. I was anxious, angry, hostile and frustrated and going up and down, really moody.

As I went through the Purification Program, I started to notice that my mood started to level off and by the end of the program I was very calm. I could have conversations with people and just sit and listen.

I ran out drugs that I had done from a lot of incidents. I became this bright person and every single sense was heightened—colors looked more vibrant and I could smell things better. I was more tuned in to sounds.

I've done a lot of amazing things, but by far this was the most amazing thing I've ever gone through, because it changed my entire life!

–T.F.

~

As a chiropractor, I know the anatomy and physiology of the body. As a former pro athlete, I was ignorant of all the negative repercussions of drugs.

I took heavy alcohol, heavy anabolic steroids to improve strength and power (of course, it hurt more than it helped), pain pills, anti-inflammatories, injections to play on, plus more street drugs: marijuana and cocaine.

Let's say, in all honesty, that getting fully rid of all the chemical cocktail residuals via the Purification Program, it truly saved my life. It's true.

Before, I had become wooden and less vital.

Now I am alive and winning much more in life.

–M.T.

~

Medical and Psychiatric Drugs

My biggest win from the Purification Program came when I was running out the effects of an antidepressant. I knew what it was because of the continual feeling of lostness and detachment. Then one night I looked up and, bang, it was gone. I mean really gone!

On my drive home I felt like a totally new person. No longer did I have that feeling of having to climb over a wall of despair in order to deal with my problems. I could now deal directly with the world and my situations without any barriers. My life is now incredible and I am totally grateful to this program for it.

–T.B.

~

I was not able to fall asleep without a sleeping pill. This made things worse in the morning; so much so, that I started taking "speed" to wake up. I then became addicted and it became a part of my daily routine.

From the day I started this program, my life has had a dramatic change for the better. I am able to go to bed at normal hours—something I was not able to do for twenty years!

The fact that I'm free from toxins and drugs has made it possible for me to enjoy life, people, places and personal emotions. I am now living for the first time in my entire life, a normal, decent, ambitious, clean, lovable and exciting life.

All this I owe to this fantastic program!

–M.E.

~

A doctor diagnosed me with a severe allergy. Every year I was in the hospital, taken to the emergency room because I'd swell up and my throat would close and I'd itch and have hives all over.

I did the Purification Program and it's amazing how much we've been affected by all these chemicals that are holding us down. I ran out all of it. And I felt so much better. Prior to this program I've never felt like I feel now.

A month went by—didn't have any symptoms, another month went by, nothing. Six months, a year and now three years later and I have never had one itch, I haven't been to the hospital and, in my eyes, I'm cured of it. It's terrific. It's absolutely great!

–K.E.

~

I thought I had a pretty light history. I didn't work around chemicals, but decided to do the program as a preventive measure.

Then, there I was, on the program sweating and all of a sudden I'm smelling medications that I took as a teenager and literally this stuff was coming out of my skin pores.

When I was done, boy, did I get the End Phenomena! I felt much better. I felt alive, I had more energy, I could think more clearly. It was just amazing. I was dancing, I was singing!

–H.W.

~

As I ran out the accumulated residues of the medications I had been given after my heart attack, I realized even more profoundly how the effects of these drugs had been holding me back. I felt myself gradually shed the drug effects, becoming more and more stable and a sense of well-being and freeness gradually surrounded me. I feel as though some cloud that I wasn't even quite aware of has lifted and my senses are once again sharp and clear.

–J.B.

~

I had a hip replacement and they had to use a large amount of morphine afterwards. When I took the morphine, I noticed that I didn't care to read or talk to people. I had no interest at all. I lost all my interest. This state continued long after I was done with the drugs and I didn't come back to normal again.

I decided to do the Purification Program and, about ten days in, all that morphine sensation came over me again and I knew that was my lucky day. It took about two days to run it all out.

When I was done with the program, I completely bounced back to my former self where I was rejuvenated in interest and enthusiasm and my desire to do things again just came back.

If I hadn't done this, I'd still be in that state of not caring and not wanting to do anything. This program saved my life!

–J.H.

~

Before the Purification Program I often felt I had no energy to do the things I loved to do. Today I'm full of a vital energy that radiates out from me! My vision has cleared as if a film has been peeled away. Colors are so much clearer and everything looks sharper. My lungs feel stronger than ever. I could smell years of asthma medications coming out of me as I sweated in the sauna. I feel healthier than I have felt in years. I feel free from years of drugs and medicines. I feel so alive! The Purification Program is the best thing I have ever done!

–T.M.

~

My doctor had told me that because of some medical tests that I've had to have, I've had a ton of radiation poured into my body. I've had anesthetics from surgeries before and I knew I wanted to clean that out. I had no idea how foggy and slow I was in life until finishing this program.

Now I look back and see the difference—it's like day and night! I always thought I was pretty fast and sharp but, wow!

My life has expanded more and more and I just continue to get brighter. It's been a few months since I finished the program and I'm doing way more than I ever was. I'm smarter. I'm sharper, I'm faster and can handle things so much better and I love it.

–J.H.

~

Following a second major operation, I had a pretty rough time. Even after initial physical recovery, I felt about ten years older, had no energy and had various pains most of the time that I never had before. I figured I'd recover and "bounce back," but this didn't happen. I kept attributing what was going on to some other reason, not the operation or the heavy painkillers that I had to take for weeks afterward.

These drugs had such a bad effect on me I decided it was better to endure the pain than the side effects. I got myself off them gradually until I stopped taking them altogether. I had a certain mental "fogginess" that persisted for a long time and I always felt not quite "there" and somewhat dizzy.

Some time later, I did the Purification Program. Through the course of the program, I gradually started to feel better and better. I then reached a point one day where I literally came out of the fog and was clearheaded, with renewed vigor and ambition. But best of all, I no longer had any pains—they were totally gone!

They have never returned, not one bit, to this day. The Purification Program literally saved my life from the effects of heavy drugs that would otherwise still be in my system, affecting my life in a major way.

–C.R.

~

I felt like I was a biochemical personality where I would fly off at the littlest thing. My temper would get the best of me and I had a hard time understanding people.

I knew something was hindering me and it was just hard to figure out. This black cloud was always around me. It was hard to think and to do things. I couldn't make up my mind.

When I got onto the Purification Program, things started to run out.

One drug that I'd taken was steroids, to handle inflammation for asthma. It has horrible side effects and as it ran out, I could feel the effect on my blood sugar and I'd get heart palpitations. Another day I was running out Tylenol—my ears were ringing and I had a little bit of the flu turning on. Then my eyes started burning as I ran out chlorine and you could smell it. I'd see tan lines from bathing suits as I ran out radiation.

I began feeling more aware and much better about myself. I understood that with drugs and toxins, if it poisons your body, it poisons you. I had more energy; I felt lighter; I felt better. I started handling things better in life. My relations with others were better. I'm more enthusiastic about life and excited to create things.

–S.M.

~

I grew up in the mid-seventies and did more than my share of experimenting with drugs while in high school. I've also had asthma since I was three years old and can't even begin to count how many bottles of inhalers I've gone through. Then I got on antidepressants and I thought that that was going to be my life.

I saw a doctor who guided me off these drugs and I got onto the Purification Program. About two weeks into it, I had a chemical smell coming off of me. It was the same kind of chemical smell from the inhalers I have. I felt like I was purging all the accumulation, the mass of drugs and toxins that had been in my system, and I felt lighter—emotionally, physically, spiritually—I felt like somebody had opened me up and I was fresh and clean inside. It is really a phenomenal feeling.

–T.M.

~

Chemical Exposure and Toxins

I've been an aircraft mechanic for over twenty years and a diesel mechanic before that. I knew I had been exposed to a lot of chemicals, solvents, adhesives and exhaust.

One of the products we've used forever is a product called Stoddard Solvent. It's got a very specific odor and it's got a very specific symptom when you have an overdose of it.

Back in the old days, we didn't wear gloves and we didn't wear respirators. You would be washing parts in the solvent tank and, after days and weeks of this, your hands would start to go numb and they would feel like they were made of rubber. You knew that it was time to get your hands out of the solvent.

Well, I haven't had my hands in solvent in seven or eight years. One day on the Purification Program I was sitting there happily sweating and I noticed my body odor had changed. I smelled Stoddard Solvent. There's nothing in the world that smells like it. And after a little while, both my hands went numb and I was suffering the effects of acute Stoddard Solvent poisoning. It lasted about a half an hour and then it went away.

It felt as if I'd taken off a backpack. I was sleeping better. I was performing better at work. I was calmer. I was more emotionally stable. It felt wonderful!

–M.M.

~

When I was much younger, I was in the Royal Air Force. I worked in a maintenance area where we cleaned pots by putting them into this big tub of carbon tetrachloride. I had no idea how powerful that stuff was. I leaned over to pick the things out of it and I was feeling dizzy and the place was spinning around and it was terrible.

I'd forgotten all about that, but while I was doing my Purification Program, there it was: the same smell and taste and everything.

Now that I'm done, my perceptions have definitely improved. I am able to actually see better and hear better and can perceive smells I wasn't aware of before. This was amazing!

−R.T.

~

I spent four years of the war in a submarine. This was an older version that ran on diesel fuel. I lived in that fuel for those years, and even when I showered I still smelled like diesel fuel. I did the Purification Program later and the results were amazing. I had complete detoxification. When I saw the chemicals come out I was totally shocked that they had stayed in my body all that time. It all just came out from my body—all the oils, fumes—gone.

−T.O.

~

I had been exposed to several toxins during the last ten years, such as mercury poisoning, construction and industrial gases and toxic mold. I hated the way I was feeling. I had mental sluggishness, my ability to recall things and make decisions had been slowed down and I couldn't think as fast as I wanted to. I wanted to get cleaned out, get my energy back and feel a lot better. I knew the Purification Program could do that.

It was just amazing. When I was done, I was able to think fast, recall much better, able to paint and write and pursue any activity I wanted to with much greater speed. It completely changed my life.

It was life-changing physically, mentally and spiritually and today, having finished a year and a half ago, I am still experiencing benefits in all those areas and I recommend this program to everybody. It's the best thing I've done.

–Y.H.

~

As a painting contractor, I was constantly exposed to toxins and painting fumes. I noticed over the years my energy level and mental clarity and focus started dropping.

As I was doing the Purification Program, I couldn't believe the amount of toxins I sweated out. You could smell the paint thinner coming out of my body.

As I did the program, I noticed my energy, my mental clarity and mental focus coming back. I don't know what I'd have done without it!

–R.S.

~

I am an artist and I have been painting for about forty-five years. I love the medium of oils, but you use turpentine and linseed oil and I didn't realize the fumes from all these chemicals were affecting me so negatively. I was starting to get discoloration in my hands and my face and having coughing spells.

About a week into my Purification Program, I was dripping in sweat and smelling turpentine and linseed oil. It was seeping out of my body! I'd get a few coughing spells and I could taste the turpentine.

I could also see paint coming out of my fingers, like burnt sienna and raw umber, and I know I paint with these, but has all that been in there?

Since I finished my program, I feel so much healthier. My thoughts are clearer and I just feel better. I started painting on a whole new level and the clarity of my thinking and everything was just so much easier. I wasn't in a fog anymore. I recommend it to every artist in every medium because we're all toxic.

–V.M.

~

As a makeup artist, I was using all sorts of products on my body and on my face and didn't realize there were actually toxic ingredients in these products.

While I was doing the Purification Program, they were running out and coming out of my body. I was getting rashes and I was itchy—I'd wipe my face and I could see it actually on the towel.

I had radiation from past sunburns, Novocain came out in my mouth, tiredness and fatigue from anesthetics from past operations, turpentine poisoning, cadmium poisoning from paint solvents and, I believe, mercury poisoning.

Since I completed the program, my life has totally changed. I don't have any more rashes, my skin is clear and the numbness in my hand is gone. I feel ambitious, I've started a new business, I feel that it saved my life.

–C.Z.

~

I have a very extensive drug history and worked with a lot of chemicals in former professions. It was very difficult for me to think clearly, which I compared to trying to locate your keys in the dark.

158

I also had a hard time concentrating and was easily distracted. My energy level was quite low and would interfere with my being able to do many of the things I wanted to do in life. I just constantly felt like sleeping.

Since completing the Purification Program, I feel like a different person. I now have much more energy for things that I really want to be doing. I find it much easier to concentrate and can mentally stay longer on a given course. I can also think much clearer and am able to solve problems with ease. Now I am able to see situations clearer, which enables me to find solutions much easier.

−E.E.

~

My first win started two to three days into the program. After the running part I noticed I could see farther, I could think a lot faster and my actions were much faster.

About the fourth day into the program, tear gas started coming out from my eyes. I was exposed to it four to five years ago and could smell it as it was coming out.

When it all ran out, I went outside and wow! Everything—my eyesight improved so much!

−V.I.

~

From the first day of taking niacin, I saw the finest sunburn reactions, with bright red knees to spider bites reappearing and then disappearing, to poison coming out from an Australian jellyfish that I encountered in the Pacific Ocean at the age of six.

As I moved on, I ran out aspirin that I'd taken to "resolve my headaches" starting when I was seven years old, to more sunburns and radiation to secondhand cigarette smoke—all of which made its way out during the course of the program.

I can simply say that I am now cleaned out, purified and am not effect of the restimulative effects of all the accumulated impurities that I had in my body. I have a fresh take on life, physically and spiritually.

–S.F.

~

In the late 1970s, I went to my doctor for a standard physical. To my horror, I was told that I had less than two years to live. He sent me to two other doctors to verify his diagnosis and they all concurred—I had arteriosclerosis. One doctor told me, "You'd better go home and write your will."

I was in despair. I was in my twenties, just newly married and it suddenly appeared that all my hopes and dreams for the future were now impossibly out of reach.

I had learned about L. Ron Hubbard's Purification Program and decided to do it, thinking that perhaps getting the built-up toxins out of my body would make things easier over the coming months.

Three weeks later, when I finished the program, I went back to my doctor for another checkup. He was absolutely astounded. He said that the results were impossible and that, even though two other doctors had verified his diagnosis, he must have been wrong because what had occurred was "medically impossible." There was no trace whatsoever of the arteriosclerosis. It was completely gone.

I have been healthy ever since. I am happily married to the same man, we have a wonderful teenage daughter and I am achieving all my hopes and dreams. I owe my life, my happiness and my success to the Purification Program.

–B.W.

~

Exposure to Hazardous Materials

World Trade Center Disaster Site

The chemical exposure suffered by first responders to the World Trade Center tragedy of 11 September 2001, is arguably among the most severe on record. Firemen, police, rescue workers and others spent months at Ground Zero, inhaling toxic fumes and dust that contained hundreds of chemicals, such as asbestos, pesticides and highly toxic components found in industrial fluids.

A facility using the program developed by L. Ron Hubbard was established near Ground Zero. From the outset the program proved remarkably effective, even for those not improving from other forms of treatment. First responders reported a range of symptoms associated with toxic-caused nerve damage—including inability to sleep, short-term memory loss, balance problems and mood swings—resolved with the program. Here is what one firefighter had to say after completing the program:

On September 11, 2001 my life, as well as the life of every other American, was turned upside down. I have been a firefighter for over nineteen years in NYC. On that horrible day I lost many of my friends as well as my brother (a firefighter), who was killed in the collapse. I spent the first many weeks digging at Ground Zero, looking for my brother and the many other victims. We were all exposed to massive amounts of toxic smoke and dust.

Over the course of three or four months after the collapse, I watched my friends, who were some of the fittest people in NYC, start getting sick with the "WTC (World Trade Center) cough." I couldn't understand why they were getting so ill. I felt very bad for them.

I had always worked out and was in excellent physical condition my whole life until 9/11. Shortly after leaving the site I began to get the same symptoms my friends had gotten earlier. I started having asthma attacks so fierce and frequent I ended up in the hospital for eight days after fighting a relatively small fire. I could only sleep two to three hours per night, with constant nightmares. I couldn't breathe without the use of inhalers. I was very fatigued and was anxious about my health and my future. My children were very concerned. I was told that my days as a firefighter were over.

After suffering for over twelve months with no real relief, I heard about the program developed by Mr. Hubbard. I jumped at the chance, as I already believed in the value of vitamins, exercise and sweating. By the third day of the program I was safely off my inhalers. I was sleeping seven to eight hours a night for the first time since 9/11 and experienced no nightmares! By day 20, I was running for twenty-five minutes and felt fantastic both physically and mentally!

My friends and family all noticed that I was looking and feeling better. My children no longer worry about whether or not I am going to live or be sick the rest of my life. I am finally back to my old self!

–J.H.
Fire Department
New York

~

The following is from the chief engineer of a building close to the World Trade Center used as the main shelter during the cleanup. He was on duty on 9/11 and remained so for weeks after the disaster.

In the months following the World Trade Center collapse, I was constantly tired and it was a struggle just to get to work every day. I had headaches all the time and was living on about ten aspirins a day just to make it through the day. It was terrible. My breathing was awful because of all the dust and I couldn't even make it up a flight of stairs without getting winded. Every day that went by, I just felt worse. I must have seen six different doctors and they gave me this and that medication and nothing seemed to work.

On my first day on the program, I was in the sauna and had a towel on my back. After a while I took a break and went out of the sauna and a few minutes later someone pointed out that my towel had turned a purple color from my sweat! That stuff was coming out of me! And for the next ten or eleven days I had stuff coming out of me every day until it just stopped. About a week after that, I had something like oil come out of my body that smelled like kerosene and left a pinkish color on the towel. These toxins were literally flushing out of my system.

After completing the program I'm about 1,000 percent better! I sleep great. I have no problems at all. I haven't had a headache since I started the program. Even my breathing has improved tremendously. My energy level is just fantastic and it feels like I am ten years younger and my mental outlook is much brighter.

I honestly feel that if I didn't do this program, if I didn't get those chemicals out of me, I was going to die within five to ten years.

–T.B.

New York City Schools

∿

Another case was a member of the Civil Service Technical Guild, which represents engineers, architects, scientists, chemists and other technical trades. The following is his report after completing the program:

More than three hundred of our members were intensively involved in the World Trade Center rescue and recovery effort and were exposed to toxic dust, smoke and fumes over a period of several months.

Many continue to suffer the effects of these exposures years after the collapse. Standard treatments are not getting to the root causes of their symptoms. Despite this, it appears that the public health response will be limited to health surveys and the hope that "Time will heal."

This program is the only treatment being offered to rescue workers that addresses the problem of toxic body burdens. I have first-hand knowledge of its efficacy.

I was quite beaten down when I arrived for treatment, not knowing what chemicals were released during the attacks or continued to be released during the rescue and recovery efforts. We may never find out all there is to know about toxic exposures that my Union members suffered in the aftermath of September 11, but I fully recovered my pre-9/11 health and job fitness.

–M.K.
Civil Service Technical Guild

~

Gulf War Syndrome

The following is but a sampling of the cases from servicemen and women who completed the program after exposure in the line of duty:

As a Gulf War veteran, the unknown toxins I was no doubt exposed to had every opportunity to wash out while I was doing the program.

I gained improved physical perception of taste and smell, greater willingness to accept my own viewpoint as it is and greater creativity. I feel more energetic, more vital and more at cause over my life.

–B.D.

~

I am a combat veteran of the Gulf War. I had been diagnosed with Persian Gulf Syndrome, also known as Gulf War Illness. My symptoms included chronic joint aches, fatigue, recurring rashes on my hands and feet, a frequent eyelid infection and short-term memory loss. Antibiotics and other prescribed and over-the-counter remedies "band-aided" some of the symptoms, but nothing completely restored me to health.

I began the program and, during my second and third days in the sauna, I had a tan-colored residue depositing with my sweat on the T-shirt and running shorts I was wearing. On about my seventeenth day on the program, I noticed a number of small black dots where my feet had been. I moved my feet to another spot on the towel and waited a minute or two. When I picked up my feet, there were more black dots. I literally had black ooze coming out of the bottom of my feet!

As I continued the program, I experienced an overall feeling of well-being, such as I had not known for many years. The joint aches were gone, the rashes were gone—in fact, all of my negative symptoms had been eliminated. I felt vibrant, alert, attentive.

When I returned home to New Hampshire, my wife and children were as amazed as I was—not only had Dad come home healthy, I was like a newer, younger version of myself! I remain symptom-free to this day.

–R.W.

~

Radiation and Radioactive Material

Numerous reports have been received that detail the results of the Purification Program on people with a history of radiation exposure.

One such case was that of a man who was among 2,100 marines who received orders to participate in early nuclear weapons testing in Nevada. He witnessed two atomic detonations. The second explosion, 77 kilotons, was the largest atmospheric blast test ever conducted within the continental limits of the United States. He was in an open trench 3 miles from the explosion. Shortly afterwards, he was sent to within 300 yards of "ground zero." His recollection of the first blast was as follows:

We were told to bend down in the ditch and cover our eyes with our forearms. When that blast went off, I could see the bone in my arm through my closed eyes. We were thrown back and forth in that ditch. It was like a stampede of cattle went over us. The force and heat were tremendous. We had burns on the backs of our necks. We weren't prepared ahead of time for any of this. We were as innocent as children until that bomb lit up the sky as bright as day and I turned to see a manikin behind me with its face on fire.

Twenty years later he started feeling sick. He said he went to thirty-six doctors, but they couldn't determine what was wrong with him. Soon after he went through the Purification Program.

My improvements were multifaceted. When I began this program, I had reached the point where I felt that a return to well-being was highly improbable if not impossible. During the first thirteen to fourteen days of the program, I continued to believe that improvement was out of the question for me. And then—WHAMO! Something miraculous happened! Damned if I didn't begin to feel better. A little better at first in subtle yet noticeable ways. For instance, my stamina increased; my feelings of tiredness began to dissipate slowly and grudgingly. Towards the end of the program I realized that I had more vitality than at any time in the last seven or eight years. Emotionally, I felt up. Depression lifted and I could once again feel exhilaration when such moments occurred. There is new hope for radiation victims! I'm the living proof of it!

–T.S.

~

The following is from another individual who was indirectly exposed to radioactive fallout from atomic tests conducted in the US.

In the very beginning of my program, something seemed to be happening that didn't make sense to me. I was starting to feel sick—I had headaches that were getting worse. I was having fevers and dry heaves. I was getting a rash on my legs. I didn't know what was going on and found out I was releasing radiation.

I was expecting radiation poisoning from the brief amount of time that I lived in Los Alamos, New Mexico (where atomic bomb testing was done), when I was an infant and that's all it took! This is what I think caused my chronic fatigue and headaches for all my life.

Once I got all the radiation out of my system, I felt great. I would wake up in the morning pain-free, which was something I didn't think would ever happen again, honestly!

When your body feels good, you have no pain, no fatigue. You start living and you get things done. I feel great!

–G.M.

~

Another individual worked on a contamination clean-up crew at the atomic research center. He had worked inside nuclear reactors and once reported inhaling highly contaminated dust. He said he recalled working in one specific area that was so "hot" he was only permitted one minute of work in the area per day. Other areas he'd worked in had longer "burn-out" time, such as ten minutes or thirty minutes. He later underwent the Purification Program.

Before the program I felt "massy" around the head. I thought I was doing okay, but I knew it wasn't quite right. I felt as though something needed to be handled. While doing the program, I went through periods of blankness for days. I just couldn't seem to remember things. Also, I went through about one week of not being able to catch my breath. You know, I didn't even realize I had had a problem with it, but now I can recall shortness of breath while mountain climbing, but only when the weather was hot. After the program, I am in great shape. I feel sharp, alert and ready to face life. I sure do feel better about life and myself now.

–B.H.

$\mathcal{A}$PPENDIX

$\mathcal{A}$PPENDIX

$\mathcal{F}$URTHER $\mathcal{S}$TUDY
BOOKS & LECTURES BY L. RON HUBBARD

The materials of Dianetics and Scientology comprise the largest body of information ever assembled on the mind, spirit and life, rigorously refined and codified by L. Ron Hubbard through five decades of research, investigation and development. The results of that work are contained in hundreds of books and more than 3,000 recorded lectures. A full listing and description of them all can be obtained from any Scientology Church or Publications Organization. (See *Guide to the Materials*.)

The books and lectures below form the foundation upon which the Bridge to Freedom is built. They are listed in the sequence Ron wrote or delivered them. In many instances, Ron gave a series of lectures immediately following the release of a new book to provide further explanation and insight of these milestones. Through monumental restoration efforts, those lectures are now available and are listed herein with their companion book.

While Ron's books contain the summaries of breakthroughs and conclusions as they appeared in the developmental research track, his lectures provide the running day-to-day record of research and explain the thoughts, conclusions, tests and demonstrations that lay along that route. In that regard, they are the complete record of the entire research track, providing not only the most important breakthroughs in Man's history, but the *why* and *how* Ron arrived at them.

Not the least advantage of a chronological study of these books and lectures is the inclusion of words and terms which, when originally used, were defined by LRH with considerable exactitude. Far beyond a mere "definition," entire lectures are devoted to a full description of each new Dianetic or Scientology term—what made the breakthrough possible, its application in auditing as well as its application to life itself. Through a sequential study, you can see how the subject progressed and recognize the highest levels of development. As a result, one leaves behind no misunderstoods, obtains a full conceptual understanding of Dianetics and Scientology and grasps the subjects at a level not otherwise possible.

This is the path to knowing how to know, unlocking the gates to your future eternity. Follow it.

DIANETICS: THE ORIGINAL THESIS • Ron's *first* description of Dianetics. Originally circulated in manuscript form, it was soon copied and passed from hand to hand. Ensuing word of mouth created such demand for more information, Ron concluded the only way to answer the inquiries was with a book. That book was Dianetics: The Modern Science of Mental Health, now the all-time self-help bestseller. Find out what started it all. For here is the bedrock foundation of Dianetic discoveries: the *Original Axioms,* the *Dynamic Principle of Existence,* the *Anatomy of the Analytical* and *Reactive Mind,* the *Dynamics,* the *Tone Scale,* the *Auditor's Code* and the first description of a *Clear.* Even more than that, here are the primary laws describing *how* and *why* auditing works. It's only here in Dianetics: The Original Thesis.

DIANETICS: THE EVOLUTION OF A SCIENCE • This is the story of *how* Ron discovered the reactive mind and developed the procedures to get rid of it. Originally written for a national magazine—published to coincide with the release of Dianetics: The Modern Science of Mental Health—it started a wildfire movement virtually overnight upon that book's publication. Here then are both the fundamentals of Dianetics as well as the only account of Ron's two-decade journey of discovery and how he applied a scientific methodology to the problems of the human mind. He wrote it so you would know. Hence, this book is a must for every Dianeticist and Scientologist.

DIANETICS: THE MODERN SCIENCE OF MENTAL HEALTH • The bolt from the blue that began a worldwide movement. For while Ron had previously announced his discovery of the reactive mind, it had only fueled the fire of those wanting more information. More to the point—it was humanly impossible for one man to clear an entire planet. Encompassing all his previous discoveries and case histories of those breakthroughs in application, Ron provided the complete handbook of Dianetics procedure to train auditors to use it everywhere. A bestseller for more than half a century, translated in more than 50 languages with tens of millions of copies in print and used in more than 100 countries of Earth, Dianetics: The Modern Science of Mental Health is, indisputably, the most widely read and influential book about the human mind ever written. And that is why it will forever be known as *Book One.*

DIANETICS LECTURES AND DEMONSTRATIONS • Immediately following the publication of *Dianetics,* LRH began lecturing to packed auditoriums across America. Although addressing thousands at a time, demand continued to grow. To meet that demand, his presentation in Oakland, California, was recorded. In these four lectures, Ron related the events that sparked his investigation and his personal journey to his groundbreaking discoveries. He followed it all with a personal demonstration of Dianetics auditing—the only such demonstration of Book One available. *4 lectures.*

176

DIANETICS PROFESSIONAL COURSE LECTURES—*A SPECIAL COURSE FOR BOOK ONE AUDITORS* • Following six months of coast-to-coast travel, lecturing to the first Dianeticists, Ron assembled auditors in Los Angeles for a new Professional Course. The subject was his next sweeping discovery on life—the *ARC Triangle*, describing the interrelationship of *Affinity, Reality* and *Communication*. Through a series of fifteen lectures, LRH announced many firsts, including the *Spectrum of Logic*, containing an infinity of gradients from right to wrong; *ARC and the Dynamics;* the *Tone Scales of ARC;* the *Auditor's Code* and how it relates to ARC; and the *Accessibility Chart* that classifies a case and how to process it. Here, then, is both the final statement on Book One Auditing Procedures and the discovery upon which all further research would advance. The data in these lectures was thought to be lost for over fifty years and only available in student notes published in Notes on the Lectures. The original recordings have now been discovered making them broadly available for the first time. Life in its highest state, *Understanding,* is composed of Affinity, Reality and Communication. And, as LRH said, the best description of the ARC Triangle to be found anywhere is in these lectures. *15 lectures.*

SCIENCE OF SURVIVAL—*PREDICTION OF HUMAN BEHAVIOR* • The most useful book you will ever own. Built around the *Hubbard Chart of Human Evaluation,* Science of Survival provides the first accurate prediction of human behavior. Included on the chart are all the manifestations of an individual's survival potential graduated from highest to lowest, making this the complete book on the Tone Scale. Knowing only one or two characteristics of a person and using this chart, you can plot his or her position on the Tone Scale and thereby know the rest, obtaining an accurate index of their *entire* personality, conduct and character. Before this book the world was convinced that cases could not improve but only deteriorate. Science of Survival presents the idea of different states of case and the brand-new idea that one can progress upward on the Tone Scale. And therein lies the basis of today's Grade Chart.

THE SCIENCE OF SURVIVAL LECTURES • Underlying the development of the Tone Scale and Chart of Human Evaluation was a monumental breakthrough: The *Theta–MEST Theory,* containing the explanation of the interaction between Life—*theta*—with the physical universe of Matter, Energy, Space and Time—*MEST*. In these lectures, delivered to students immediately following publication of the book, Ron gave the most expansive description of all that lies behind the Chart of Human Evaluation and its application in life itself. Moreover, here also is the explanation of how the ratio of *theta* and *en(turbulated)-theta* determines one's position on the Tone Scale and the means to ascend to higher states. *6 lectures.*

177

SELF ANALYSIS • The barriers of life are really just shadows. Learn to know yourself—not just a shadow of yourself. Containing the most complete description of consciousness, Self Analysis takes you through your past, through your potentials, your life. First, with a series of self-examinations and using a special version of the Hubbard Chart of Human Evaluation, you plot yourself on the Tone Scale. Then, applying a series of light yet powerful processes, you embark on the great adventure of self-discovery. This book further contains embracive principles that reach *any* case, from the lowest to the highest—including auditing techniques so effective they are referred to by Ron again and again through all following years of research into the highest states. In sum, this book not only moves one up the Tone Scale but can pull a person out of almost anything.

ADVANCED PROCEDURE AND AXIOMS • With new breakthroughs on the nature and anatomy of engrams—"Engrams are effective only when the individual himself determines that they will be effective"—came the discovery of the being's use of a *Service Facsimile:* a mechanism employed to explain away failures in life, but which then locks a person into detrimental patterns of behavior and further failure. In consequence came a new type of processing addressing *Thought, Emotion* and *Effort* detailed in the "Fifteen Acts" of Advanced Procedure and oriented to the rehabilitation of the preclear's *Self-determinism.* Hence, this book also contains the all-encompassing, no-excuses-allowed explanation of *Full Responsibility,* the key to unlocking it all. Moreover, here is the codification of *Definitions, Logics,* and *Axioms,* providing both the summation of the entire subject and direction for all future research. *See Handbook for Preclears, written as a companion self-processing manual to Advanced Procedure and Axioms.*

> **THOUGHT, EMOTION AND EFFORT** • With the codification of the Axioms came the means to address key points on a case that could unravel all aberration. *Basic Postulates, Prime Thought, Cause and Effect* and their effect on everything from *memory* and *responsibility* to an individual's own role in empowering *engrams*—these matters are only addressed in this series. Here, too, is the most complete description of the *Service Facsimile* found anywhere—and why its resolution removes an individual's self-imposed disabilities. *21 lectures.*

HANDBOOK FOR PRECLEARS • The "Fifteen Acts" of Advanced Procedure and Axioms are paralleled by the fifteen Self-processing Acts given in Handbook for Preclears. Moreover, this book contains several essays giving the most expansive description of the *Ideal State of Man*. Discover why behavior patterns become so solidly fixed; why habits seemingly can't be broken; how decisions long ago have more power over a person than his decisions today; and why a person keeps past negative experiences in the present. It's all clearly laid out on the Chart of Attitudes—a milestone breakthrough that complements the Chart of Human Evaluation—plotting the ideal state of being and one's *attitudes* and *reactions* to life. *In self-processing, Handbook for Preclears is used in conjunction with Self Analysis.*

THE LIFE CONTINUUM • Besieged with requests for lectures on his latest breakthroughs, Ron replied with everything they wanted and more at the Second Annual Conference of Dianetic Auditors. Describing the technology that lies behind the self-processing steps of the *Handbook*—here is the *how* and *why* of it all: the discovery of *Life Continuum*—the mechanism by which an individual is compelled to carry on the life of another deceased or departed individual, generating in his own body the infirmities and mannerisms of the departed. Combined with auditor instruction on use of the Chart of Attitudes in determining how to enter every case at the proper gradient, here, too, are directions for dissemination of the Handbook and hence, the means to begin wide-scale clearing. *10 lectures.*

SCIENTOLOGY: MILESTONE ONE • Ron began the first lecture in this series with six words that would change the world forever: "This is a course in *Scientology*." From there, Ron not only described the vast scope of this, a then brand-new subject, he also detailed his discoveries on past lives. He proceeded from there to the description of the first E-Meter and its initial use in uncovering the *theta line* (the entire track of a thetan's existence), as entirely distinct from the *genetic body line* (the time track of bodies and their physical evolution), shattering the "one-life" lie and revealing the *whole track* of spiritual existence. Here, then, is the very genesis of Scientology. *22 lectures.*

THE ROUTE TO INFINITY: TECHNIQUE 80 LECTURES • As Ron explained, "Technique 80 is the *To Be or Not To Be* Technique." With that, he unveiled the crucial foundation on which ability and sanity rest: *the being's capacity to make a decision.* Here, then, is the anatomy of "maybe," the *Wavelengths of ARC,* the *Tone Scale of Decisions,* and the means to rehabilitate a being's ability *To Be*... almost *anything. 7 lectures. (Knowledge of Technique 80 is required for Technique 88 as described in Scientology: A History of Man—below.)*

SCIENTOLOGY: A HISTORY OF MAN • "A cold-blooded and factual account of your last 76 trillion years." So begins A History of Man, announcing the revolutionary *Technique 88*—revealing for the first time the truth about whole track experience and the exclusive address, in auditing, to the thetan. Here is history unraveled with the first E-Meter, delineating and describing the principal incidents on the whole track to be found in any human being: *Electronic implants, entities,* the *genetic track, between-lives incidents, how bodies evolved* and *why you got trapped in them*—they're all detailed here.

    TECHNIQUE 88: INCIDENTS ON THE TRACK BEFORE EARTH • "Technique 88 is the most hyperbolical, effervescent, dramatic, unexaggeratable, high-flown, superlative, grandiose, colossal and magnificent technique which the mind of Man could conceivably embrace. It is as big as the whole track and all the incidents on it. It's what you apply it to; it's what's been going on. It contains the riddles and secrets, the mysteries of all time. You could bannerline this technique like they do a sideshow, but nothing you could say, no adjective you could use, would adequately describe even a small segment of it. It not only batters the imagination, it makes you ashamed to imagine anything," is Ron's introduction to you in this never-before-available lecture series, expanding on all else contained in History of Man. What awaits you is the whole track itself. *15 lectures.*

SCIENTOLOGY 8-80 • The *first* explanation of the electronics of human thought and the energy phenomena in any being. Discover how even physical universe laws of motion are mirrored in a being, not to mention the electronics of aberration. Here is the link between theta and MEST revealing what energy *is*, and how you *create* it. It was this breakthrough that revealed the subject of a thetan's *flows* and which, in turn, is applied in *every* auditing process today. In the book's title, "8-8" stands for *Infinity-Infinity,* and "0" represents the static, *theta*. Included are the *Wavelengths of Emotion, Aesthetics, Beauty and Ugliness, Inflow and Outflow* and the *Sub-zero Tone Scale*—applicable only to the thetan.

    SOURCE OF LIFE ENERGY • Beginning with the announcement of his new book—Scientology 8-80—Ron not only unveiled his breakthroughs of theta as the Source of Life Energy, but detailed the *Methods of Research* he used to make that and every other discovery of Dianetics and Scientology: the *Qs* and *Logics*—methods of *thinking* applicable to any universe or thinking process. Here, then, is both *how to think* and *how to evaluate all data and knowledge,* and thus, the linchpin to a full understanding of both Scientology and life itself. *14 lectures.*

THE COMMAND OF THETA • While in preparation of his newest book and the Doctorate Course he was about to deliver, Ron called together auditors for a new Professional Course. As he said, "For the first time with this class we are stepping, really, beyond the scope of the word *Survival*." From that vantage point, the Command of Theta gives the technology that bridges the knowledge from 8-80 to 8-8008, and provides the first full explanation of the subject of *Cause* and a permanent shift of orientation in life from MEST to *Theta*. *10 lectures.*

SCIENTOLOGY 8-8008 • The complete description of the behavior and potentials of a *thetan,* and textbook for the Philadelphia Doctorate Course and The Factors: Admiration and the Renaissance of Beingness lectures. As Ron said, the book's title serves to fix in the mind of the individual a route by which he can rehabilitate himself, his abilities, his ethics and his goals—the attainment of *infinity* (8) by the reduction of the apparent *infinity* (8) of the MEST universe to *zero* (0) and the increase of the apparent *zero* (0) of one's own universe to *infinity* (8). Condensed herein are more than 80,000 hours of investigation, with a summarization and amplification of every breakthrough to date—and the full significance of those discoveries form the new vantage point of *Operating Thetan.*

THE PHILADELPHIA DOCTORATE COURSE LECTURES • This renowned series stands as the largest single body of work on the anatomy, behavior and potentials of the spirit of Man ever assembled, providing the very fundamentals which underlie the route to Operating Thetan. Here it is in complete detail—the thetan's relationship to the *creation, maintenance* and *destruction of universes.* In just those terms, here is the *anatomy* of matter, energy, space and time, and *postulating* universes into existence. Here, too, is the thetan's fall from whole track abilities and the *universal laws* by which they are restored. In short, here is Ron's codification of the upper echelon of theta beingness and behavior. Lecture after lecture fully expands every concept of the course text, Scientology 8-8008, providing the total scope of *you* in native state. *76 lectures and accompanying reproductions of the original 54 LRH hand-drawn lecture charts.*

THE FACTORS: ADMIRATION AND THE RENAISSANCE OF BEINGNESS • With the *potentials* of a thetan fully established came a look outward resulting in Ron's monumental discovery of a *universal solvent* and the basic laws of the theta *universe*—laws quite literally senior to anything: *The Factors: Summation of the Considerations of the Human Spirit and Material Universe.* So dramatic were these breakthroughs, Ron expanded the book Scientology 8-8008, both clarifying previous discoveries and adding chapter after chapter which, studied with these lectures, provide a postgraduate level to the Doctorate Course. Here then are lectures containing the knowledge of *universal truth* unlocking the riddle of creation itself. *18 lectures.*

THE CREATION OF HUMAN ABILITY—*A HANDBOOK FOR SCIENTOLOGISTS* • On the heels of his discoveries of Operating Thetan came a year of intensive research, exploring the realm of a *thetan exterior*. Through auditing and instruction, including 450 lectures in this same twelve-month span, Ron codified the entire subject of Scientology. And it's all contained in this handbook, from a *Summary of Scientology* to its basic *Axioms* and *Codes*. Moreover, here is *Intensive Procedure,* containing the famed Exteriorization Processes of *Route 1* and *Route 2*—processes drawn right from the Axioms. Each one is described in detail—*how* the process is used, *why* it works, the axiomatic technology that underlies its use, and the complete explanation of how a being can break the *false agreements* and *self-created barriers* that enslave him to the physical universe. In short, this book contains the ultimate summary of thetan exterior OT ability and its permanent accomplishment.

PHOENIX LECTURES: FREEING THE HUMAN SPIRIT • Here is the panoramic view of Scientology complete. Having codified the subject of Scientology in Creation of Human Ability, Ron then delivered a series of half-hour lectures to specifically accompany a full study of the book. From the *essentials* that underlie the technology—*The Axioms, Conditions of Existence* and *Considerations and Mechanics,* to the processes of *Intensive Procedure,* including twelve lectures describing one-by-one the thetan exterior processes of *Route 1*—it's all covered in full, providing a conceptual understanding of the *science of knowledge* and *native state OT ability.* Here then are the bedrock principles upon which everything in Scientology rests, including the embracive statement of the religion and its heritage—*Scientology, Its General Background.* Hence, this is the watershed lecture series on Scientology itself, and the axiomatic foundation for all future research. *42 lectures.*

DIANETICS 55!—*THE COMPLETE MANUAL OF HUMAN COMMUNICATION* • With all breakthroughs to date, a single factor had been isolated as crucial to success in every type of auditing. As LRH said, "Communication is so thoroughly important today in Dianetics and Scientology (as it always has been on the whole track) that it could be said if you were to get a preclear into communication, you would get him well." And this book delineates the *exact,* but previously unknown, anatomy and formulas for *perfect* communication. The magic of the communication cycle is *the* fundamental of auditing and the primary reason auditing works. The breakthroughs here opened new vistas of application—discoveries of such magnitude, LRH called Dianetics 55! the *Second Book* of Dianetics.

THE UNIFICATION CONGRESS: COMMUNICATION! FREEDOM & ABILITY • The historic Congress announcing the reunification of the subjects of Dianetics and Scientology with the release of *Dianetics 55!* Until now, each had operated in their own sphere: Dianetics addressed Man *as Man*—the first four dynamics, while Scientology addressed *life itself*—the Fifth to Eighth Dynamics. The formula which would serve as the foundation for all future development was contained in a single word: *Communication.* It was a paramount breakthrough Ron would later call, "the great discovery of Dianetics and Scientology." Here, then, are the lectures, as it happened. *16 lectures and accompanying reproductions of the original LRH hand-drawn lecture charts.*

SCIENTOLOGY: THE FUNDAMENTALS OF THOUGHT—*THE BASIC BOOK OF THE THEORY AND PRACTICE OF SCIENTOLOGY FOR BEGINNERS* • Designated by Ron as the *Book One of Scientology*. After having fully unified and codified the subjects of Dianetics and Scientology came the refinement of their *fundamentals*. Originally published as a résumé of Scientology for use in translations into non-English tongues, this book is of inestimable value to both the beginner and advanced student of the mind, spirit and life. Equipped with this book alone, one can begin a practice and perform seeming miracle changes in the states of well-being, ability and intelligence of people. Contained within are the *Conditions of Existence, Eight Dynamics, ARC Triangle, Parts of Man*, the full analysis of *Life as a Game*, and more, including exact processes for individual application of these principles in processing. Here, then, in one book, is the starting point for bringing Scientology to people everywhere.

HUBBARD PROFESSIONAL COURSE LECTURES • While Fundamentals of Thought stands as an introduction to the subject for beginners, it also contains a distillation of fundamentals for every Scientologist. Here are the in-depth descriptions of those fundamentals, each lecture one-half hour in length and providing, one-by-one, a complete mastery of a single Scientology breakthrough—*Axioms 1–10; The Anatomy of Control; Handling of Problems; Start, Change and Stop; Confusion and Stable Data; Exteriorization; Valences* and more—the *why* behind them, *how* they came to be and their mechanics. And it's all brought together with the *Code of a Scientologist*, point by point, and its use in actually creating a new civilization. In short, here are the LRH lectures that make a *Professional Scientologist*—one who can apply the subject to every aspect of life. *21 lectures.*

$\mathcal{A}$DDITIONAL BOOKS CONTAINING SCIENTOLOGY ESSENTIALS

WORK

THE PROBLEMS OF WORK—*SCIENTOLOGY APPLIED TO THE WORKADAY WORLD* • Having codified the entire subject of Scientology, Ron immediately set out to provide the *beginning* manual for its application by anyone. As he described it: life is composed of seven-tenths work, one-tenth familial, one-tenth political and one-tenth relaxation. Here, then, is Scientology applied to that seven-tenths of existence including the answers to *Exhaustion* and the *Secret of Efficiency*. Here, too, is the analysis of life itself—a game composed of exact rules. Know them and you succeed. Problems of Work contains technology no one can live without, and that can immediately be applied by both the Scientologist and those new to the subject.

LIFE PRINCIPLES

SCIENTOLOGY: A NEW SLANT ON LIFE • Scientology essentials for every aspect of life. Basic answers that put you in charge of your existence, truths to consult again and again: *Is It Possible to Be Happy?, Two Rules for Happy Living, Personal Integrity, The Anti-Social Personality* and many more. In every part of this book you will find Scientology truths that describe conditions in your life and furnish *exact* ways to improve them. Scientology: A New Slant on Life contains essential knowledge for every Scientologist and a perfect introduction for anyone new to the subject.

AXIOMS, CODES AND SCALES

SCIENTOLOGY 0-8: THE BOOK OF BASICS • The companion to *all* Ron's books, lectures and materials. This is *the* Book of Basics, containing indispensable data you will refer to constantly: the *Axioms of Dianetics and Scientology; The Factors;* a full compilation of all *Scales*—more than 100 in all; listings of the *Perceptics* and *Awareness Levels;* all *Codes* and *Creeds* and much more. The senior laws of existence are condensed into this single volume, distilled from more than 15,000 pages of writings, 3,000 lectures and scores of books.

SCIENTOLOGY ETHICS:
TECHNOLOGY OF OPTIMUM SURVIVAL

INTRODUCTION TO SCIENTOLOGY ETHICS • A new hope for Man arises with the first workable technology of ethics—technology to help an individual pull himself out of the downward skid of life and to a higher plateau of survival. This is the comprehensive handbook providing the crucial fundamentals: *Basics of Ethics & Justice; Honesty; Conditions of Existence; Condition Formulas* from Confusion to Power; the *Basics of Suppression* and its handling; as well as *Justice Procedures* and their use in Scientology Churches. Here, then, is the technology to overcome any barriers in life and in one's personal journey up the Bridge to Total Freedom.

PURIFICATION

CLEAR BODY, CLEAR MIND—*THE EFFECTIVE PURIFICATION PROGRAM* • *(This current volume.)* We live in a biochemical world, and this book is the solution. While investigating the harmful effects that earlier drug use had on preclears' cases, Ron made the major discovery that many street drugs, particularly LSD, remained in a person's body long after ingested. Residues of the drug, he noted, could have serious and lasting effects, including triggering further "trips." Additional research revealed that a wide range of substances—medical drugs, alcohol, pollutants, household chemicals and even food preservatives—could also lodge in the body's tissues. Through research on thousands of cases, he developed the *Purification Program* to eliminate their destructive effects. Clear Body, Clear Mind details every aspect of the all-natural regimen that can free one from the harmful effects of drugs and other toxins, opening the way for spiritual progress.

WHAT IS SCIENTOLOGY?

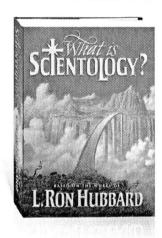

The complete and essential encyclopedic reference on the subject and practice of Scientology. Organized for use, this book contains the pertinent data on every aspect of the subject:

- The life of L. Ron Hubbard and his path of discovery
- The Spiritual Heritage of the religion
- A full description of Dianetics and Scientology
- Auditing—what it is and how it works
- Courses—what they contain and how they are structured
- The Grade Chart of Services and how one ascends to higher states
- The Scientology Ethics and Justice System
- The Organizational Structure of the Church
- A complete description of the many Social Betterment programs supported by the Church, including: Drug Rehabilitation, Criminal Reform, Literacy and Education and the instilling of real values for morality

Over 1,000 pages in length, with more than 500 photographs and illustrations, this text further includes Creeds, Codes, a full listing of all books and materials as well as a Catechism with answers to virtually any question regarding the subject.

You Ask and This Book Answers.

THE SCIENTOLOGY HANDBOOK

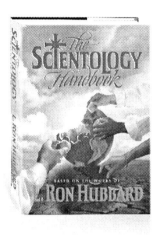

Scientology fundamentals for daily use in every part of life. Encompassing 19 separate bodies of technology, here is the most comprehensive manual on the basics of life ever published. Each chapter contains key principles and technology for your continual use:

- Study Technology
- The Dynamics of Existence
- The Components of Understanding—Affinity, Reality and Communication
- The Tone Scale
- Communication and its Formulas
- Assists for Illnesses and Injuries
- How to Resolve Conflicts
- Integrity and Honesty
- Ethics and Condition Formulas
- Answers to Suppression and a Dangerous Environment
- Marriage
- Children
- Tools for the Workplace

More than 700 photographs and illustrations make it easy for you to learn the procedures and apply them at once. This book is truly the indispensable handbook for every Scientologist.

The Technology to Build a Better World.

THE
L. RON HUBBARD
SERIES

T o really know life," L. Ron Hubbard wrote, "you've got to be part of life. You must get down and look, you must get into the nooks and crannies of existence. You have to rub elbows with all kinds and types of men before you can finally establish what he is."

Through his long and extraordinary journey to the founding of Dianetics and Scientology, Ron did just that. From his adventurous youth in a rough and tumble American West to his far-flung trek across a still mysterious Asia; from his two-decade search for the very essence of life to the triumph of Dianetics and Scientology—such are the stories recounted in the L. Ron Hubbard Biographical Publications.

Presenting the photographic overview of Ron's greater journey is *L. Ron Hubbard: Images of a Lifetime*. Drawn from his own archival collection, this is Ron's life as he himself saw it.

While for the many aspects of that rich and varied life, stands the L. Ron Hubbard Series. Each issue focuses on a specific LRH profession: *Humanitarian, Philosopher, Poet, Music Maker, Photographer* and many more including his published articles on *Freedom* and his personal *Letters & Journals*. Here is the life of a man who lived at least twenty lives in the space of one.

FOR FURTHER INFORMATION VISIT
www.lronhubbard.org

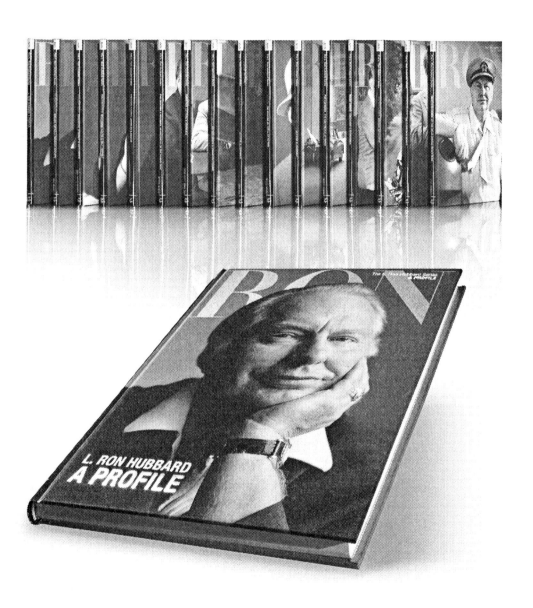

GUIDE TO THE MATERIALS

YOU'RE ON AN ADVENTURE! HERE'S THE MAP.

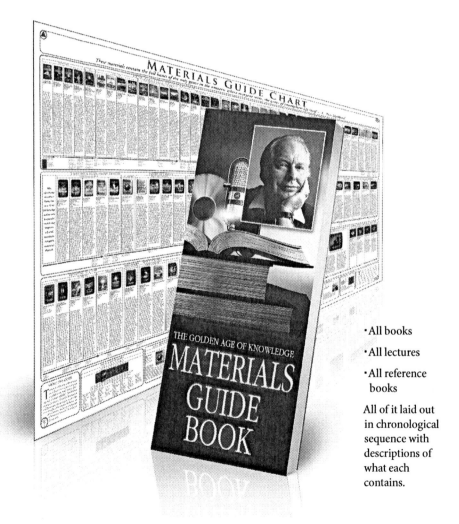

- All books
- All lectures
- All reference books

All of it laid out in chronological sequence with descriptions of what each contains.

*Y*our journey to a full understanding of Dianetics and Scientology is the greatest adventure of all. But you need a map that shows you where you are and where you are going.

That map is the Materials Guide Chart. It shows all Ron's books and lectures with a full description of their content and subject matter so you can find exactly what *you* are looking for and precisely what *you* need.

Since each book and lecture is laid out in chronological sequence, you can see *how* the subjects of Dianetics and Scientology were developed. And what that means is by simply studying this chart you are in for cognition after cognition!

New editions of all books include extensive glossaries, containing definitions for every technical term. And as a result of a monumental restoration program, the entire library of Ron's lectures are now available on compact disc, with complete transcripts, glossaries, lecture graphs, diagrams and issues he refers to in the lectures. As a result, you get *all* the data, and can learn with ease, gaining a full *conceptual* understanding.

And what that adds up to is a new Golden Age of Knowledge every Dianeticist and Scientologist has dreamed of.

To obtain your FREE Materials Guide Chart and Book, or to order L. Ron Hubbard's books and lectures, contact:

US AND INTERNATIONAL:
Bridge Publications, Inc.
5600 E. Olympic Boulevard
Commerce, California 90022
www.bridgepub.com
Phone: 1-800-722-1733
Fax: 1-323-888-6202

UNITED KINGDOM AND EUROPE:
New Era Publications International ApS
Smedeland 20
2600 Glostrup, Denmark
www.newerapublications.com
Phone: +800-808-8-8008
Fax: (45) 33 73 66 89

Books and lectures are also available direct from Churches of Scientology.
See ***Addresses***.

ADDRESSES

S cientology is the fastest-growing religion in the world today. Churches and Missions exist in cities throughout the world, and new ones are continually forming.

To obtain more information or to locate the Church nearest you, visit the Scientology website:

www.scientology.org
e-mail: info@scientology.org

or

Phone: 1-800-334-LIFE
(for US and Canada)

You can also write to any one of the Publications Organizations, listed on the following page, who can direct you to one of the thousands of Churches and Missions world over.

L. Ron Hubbard's books and lectures may be obtained from any of these addresses or direct from the publishers on the previous page.

PUBLICATIONS ORGANIZATIONS:

UNITED STATES

BRIDGE PUBLICATIONS, INC.
5600 E. Olympic Boulevard
Commerce, California 90022
info@bridgepub.com

CANADA

**CONTINENTAL PUBLICATIONS
LIAISON OFFICE CANADA**
793435 3rd Line
Mono EHS, Orangeville
Ontario L9W 2Y8
Canada
info@scientology.ca

LATIN AMERICA

**CONTINENTAL PUBLICATIONS
LIAISON OFFICE LATIN AMERICA**
Era Dinamica Editores
S.A. de C.V.
Fuente de Anahuac 1
Colonia Lomas de las Palmas
C.P. 52788, Huixquilucan
Estado de Mexico
Mexico
info@scientology.org.mx

UNITED KINGDOM

**CONTINENTAL PUBLICATIONS
LIAISON OFFICE
UNITED KINGDOM**
NEW ERA Publications
United Kingdom Ltd.
Saint Hill Manor
East Grinstead, West Sussex
England, RH19 4JY
info@scientology.org.uk

EUROPE

**NEW ERA PUBLICATIONS
INTERNATIONAL ApS**
Smedeland 20
2600 Glostrup
Denmark
info@newerapublications.com

AFRICA

**CONTINENTAL PUBLICATIONS
LIAISON OFFICE AFRICA**
Continental Publications Pty Ltd.
5 Cynthia Street
Kensington
Johannesburg 2094
South Africa
info@scientology.org.za

AUSTRALIA, NEW ZEALAND & OCEANIA

**CONTINENTAL PUBLICATIONS
LIAISON OFFICE ANZO**
NEW ERA Publications Australia Pty Ltd.
20 Dorahy Street
Dundas
New South Wales 2117
Australia
info@scientology.org.au

$\mathcal{B}$ECOME A MEMBER
OF THE INTERNATIONAL
ASSOCIATION OF SCIENTOLOGISTS

$\mathcal{T}$he International Association of Scientologists is the membership organization of all Scientologists united in the most vital crusade on Earth.

A free Six-Month Introductory Membership is extended to anyone who has not held a membership with the Association before.

As a member, you are eligible for discounts on Scientology materials offered only to IAS Members. You also receive the Association magazine, *IMPACT,* issued six times a year, full of Scientology news from around the world.

The purpose of the IAS is:

"To unite, advance, support and protect Scientology and Scientologists in all parts of the world so as to achieve the Aims of Scientology as originated by L. Ron Hubbard."

Join the strongest force for positive change on the planet today, opening the lives of millions to the greater truth embodied in Scientology.

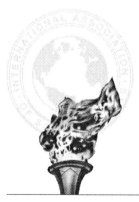

JOIN THE INTERNATIONAL
ASSOCIATION OF SCIENTOLOGISTS.

To apply for membership,
write to the International
Association of Scientologists
c/o Saint Hill Manor, East Grinstead
West Sussex, England, RH19 4JY

www.iasmembership.org

$\mathcal{E}$DITOR'S GLOSSARY
OF WORDS, TERMS AND PHRASES

Words often have several meanings. The definitions used here only give the meaning that the word has as it is used in this book. Beside each definition you will find the page on which it first appears, so you can refer back to the text if you wish.

This glossary is not meant to take the place of standard language dictionaries, which should be referred to for any words, terms or phrases that do not appear below.

–The Editor

abound: occur or exist in great quantities or numbers. Page 8.

absorption: the passage of material into the body, as by entering through the pores of the skin. Page 70.

abundance: a large quantity that is more than enough. Page 8.

abuse(s): the use of something in a way that is illegal, improper or harmful. Page 49.

acceleration: increase in how fast something happens. Page 10.

accordingly: in alignment with what has been said. Page 117.

account, taking into: considering or including a specified thing along with other factors before taking action. Page 80.

accustomed to: used to; in the habit of. Page 11.

acidic: being or containing an *acid,* any of a large class of sour-tasting, corrosive substances. There are many different acids of varying strengths, such as lemon juice and vinegar, and stronger solutions, such as the acid in a car battery. Page 66.

acute: severe and brief, as opposed to chronic (long-lasting; said of a condition that lasts over a long period). Page 155.

197

adage: a traditional saying that expresses something taken as a general truth. Page 108.

addiction: the condition of taking harmful drugs and being unable to stop taking them. Page 9.

additive(s): 1. substances added directly to food during processing, as for preservation or to change its texture or color. Page 13.
2. something needless or harmful which has been done in addition to standard procedure. Page 50.

addressed: concerned, involved with or directed to. Page 9.

adequate(ly): enough in quantity, or good enough in quality, for a particular purpose or need. Page 40.

adhered to: (of rules or instructions) followed exactly. Page 33.

administer: provide, give or supply. Page i.

adverse(ly): creating results that are harmful. Page 19.

advisable: recommended, desirable or wise, as a course of action. Page 38.

advised: 1. recommended or suggested. Page 41.
2. informed or given notice to someone for consideration of something as a course of action, decision, etc. Page 109.

aftermath: something that results or follows from an event, especially one of a disastrous or unfortunate nature. Page 166.

agent(s): something such as a chemical substance, organism or natural force that causes an effect, as in a cleansing agent. Page 8.

agonizing: causing great pain or suffering. Page 95.

agony: extreme physical or mental pain. Page 96.

agricultural: of or having to do with *agriculture,* the occupation, business or science of cultivating the land, producing crops and raising animals for food. Page 9.

alkaline: having the properties of or containing an *alkali,* a solid, liquid or gas that usually dissolves in water. Baking soda, soap and detergent all make alkaline solutions when dissolved in water. When an alkali is mixed with an acid, the acid becomes neutral. Page 66.

allergy(ies): a condition whereby a person has an unusual sensitivity to a normally harmless substance that, when breathed in, ingested or brought into contact with the skin, provokes a strong reaction from the person's body. Page 55.

all manner of: many different kinds of; all sorts of. Page 100.

all too: quite; altogether. Used to emphasize that something is the case to an extreme or unwelcome extent. Page 11.

anabolic steroids: also called *steroids,* drugs that promote muscle and bone growth (from *anabolism,* the process in the body of building body tissues). Steroids are used in medicine to promote healing, but when used for nonmedical purposes by athletes to temporarily increase the size of their muscles, these drugs are considered dangerous and are banned. Page 149.

anemia: a condition in which the number of healthy red blood cells falls below normal. Red blood cells pick up oxygen in the lungs and carry it to tissues throughout the body. In an anemic person the blood cannot provide the tissues with enough oxygen. Thus the person feels weak or tired or experiences shortness of breath. Page 33.

anemic: having anemia. *See also* **anemia.** Page 33.

anesthetic(s): a drug that reduces sensitivity to pain and may produce unconsciousness when used for major surgery. Page 40.

anesthetized: deprived of sensation; incapable of feeling. Page 96.

antibiotics: substances that are able to kill or inactivate bacteria in the body. Antibiotics are derived from microorganisms (very small living organisms) or are synthetically produced. Page 167.

antidepressant(s): the name given to a class of drugs prescribed by psychiatrists and physicians as a solution for "depression" (the label given to describe sadness or emotional withdrawal) and expanded to include a wide range of symptoms, from decreased appetite to fatigue. Antidepressants deaden one's emotions and often bring about a highly agitated state. Some of the side effects include not only dizziness, fainting, severe headaches, raised blood pressure, difficulty sleeping and interference with sexual function, but also homicidal and suicidal thoughts and behavior. Page 149.

anti-inflammatories: medications that act to reduce certain signs of inflammation, as swelling, tenderness, fever and pain. For example, aspirin is a type of anti-inflammatory. Page 149.

anxiety: feelings of worry, nervousness or concern, especially about something that is about to happen. Page 25.

apparel: a person's clothing. Page 38.

apparent: capable of being easily perceived by the senses or understanding as certainly existing or present. Page 19.

appendix: a section giving extra information at the end of a book or document. Page 173.

apt to: likely to; inclined to. Page i.

arguably: in a way that can be supported or proved with evidence and with convincing arguments. Page 163.

arsenic: a silvery-white, brittle, very poisonous chemical element. It is used in a wide range of products from glass and lead to military poison gases and insecticides. It is most commonly lethal in large doses, but repeated inhalation of the gases or dust can also be fatal because these accumulate in the body. Page 10.

arteriosclerosis: a disease of the arteries (tubes that carry blood away from the heart) involving an abnormal thickening and hardening (loss of elasticity) of the walls of the arteries, often present in old age. Page 160.

asbestos: a mineral that was used in building construction until it was discovered to be a cause of certain cancers. Asbestos has been used for insulation and fireproofing because of its heat-resistant properties. Page 12.

aspect(s): one side or part of something; a phase or part of a whole. Page 24.

aspirin: a drug used to reduce pain, fever and swelling. Page 107.

asthma: a chronic disorder characterized by wheezing, coughing, difficulty in breathing and a suffocating feeling, usually caused by an allergy. Page 152.

astound: overwhelm with amazement; surprise greatly. Page 160.

at large: as a whole; in general; (taken) altogether. Page 9.

atmospheric poisons: poisons that exist in the air of a particular place. An example of an atmospheric poison would be a toxic chemical ejected into the air of a town from a factory, poisoning the atmosphere for all those in the town. Page 7.

atomic: having to do with atomic energy, which is produced when the central part of an atom (nucleus) splits apart. The pieces of the nucleus then strike other nuclei (centers of atoms) and cause them to split, thus creating a chain reaction accompanied by a significant release of energy. Atomic bombs, as used in an atomic war, produce atomic energy. There is another type of atomic energy produced in power plants. Although the energy is used for good purposes, it can be highly dangerous to those working in the plants if a leak occurs. Page 14.

atomic bomb: an extremely destructive type of bomb, the power of which results from the immense quantity of energy suddenly released with the splitting of the nuclei (centers) of atoms into fragments. Page 169.

atrophy: shrinking or weakening of some organ or body part, usually caused by injury, disease or lack of use. Page 10.

"attention deficit": a psychiatric label applied to persons (mainly children) who are viewed as having a deficit (lack) in the ability to focus attention. *See also* **Ritalin.** Page 103.

autopsy(ies): the medical examination of a dead body to establish the cause and circumstances of death. Page 22.

back of: behind; with a hidden background relation, as in what exists behind and in support of something. Page 65.

bacterial: consisting of, caused by or connected with *bacteria,* single-celled microorganisms (organisms that can be seen only under a microscope), some of which can cause infectious diseases. Page 47.

band-aided: served as a makeshift, limited or temporary aid or solution. It is a figurative use of the brand name of an adhesive bandage with a gauze pad in the center, employed to protect minor wounds. Page 167.

B complex (vitamin): a group of water-soluble vitamins found in yeast, eggs, liver and vegetables, essential in normal body growth and nerve function. Page 45.

bear out: prove something to be true; confirm. Page 14.

behavioral: having to do with the way in which an individual acts or conducts himself or herself. Page 19.

beneficial: improving a situation; helpful, useful or favorable. Page 53.

best of, get the: defeat somebody in some way or be more than somebody can control. Page 153.

better, for the: in a way that improves a person, situation or condition. Page 150.

better, had: it would be wise to do something. Page 61.

biochemical: the interaction of life forms and chemical substances. *Bio-* means life; of living things. From the Greek *bios,* life or way of life. *Chemical* means of or having to do with *chemicals,* substances, simple or complex, that are the building blocks of matter. Page 7.

biochemical personality: an artificial personality, one that is changed (on account of biochemical factors) from the person's original personality to one secretly harboring hostilities and hatreds he does not permit to show on the surface. *Biochemical* means the interaction of life forms and chemical substances. Page 153.

biochemist: a person trained in and who practices *biochemistry,* the scientific study of the chemical substances, processes and reactions that occur in living organisms. Page 55.

biochemistry: 1. the chemical properties, reactions and phenomena of living matter. Page 22.
2. the scientific study of the chemical substances, processes and reactions that occur in living organisms. Page 45.

biophysical: of or relating to the application of methods of improving a person's ability to handle his body and environment. Page 27.

Bioplasma: the brand name for cell salts, created by biochemist Dr. William Schuessler, who in 1873 established a formula of twelve mineral combinations the body uses, in proper balance, in all of its cells. These minerals aid in the normal functioning and health of bodily tissues. Cell salts are commonly taken in the form of tablets that dissolve under the tongue. Page 41.

blast: an explosion of a bomb; also the accompanying *blast wave,* the highly compressed air that is like a wall moving rapidly away from the *fireball,* the cloud of dust and extremely hot gases created when the bomb explodes. Violent winds and intense

radiation and heat accompany the blast. *See also* **Nevada.**
Page 168.

blew: vanished or disappeared, in reference to an unwanted physical or mental sensation that suddenly went away, with an accompanying feeling of relief. Page 79.

block off: put up or form a barrier that prevents something from being felt. Page 95.

blood sugar: the level, amount or concentration of glucose in the blood. *Glucose* is a simple sugar which is an important energy source in living organisms. A blood sugar level that is higher than normal can cause harm to the nerves that control heart rate, sometimes resulting in too fast a heartbeat. Page 154.

bluntly: in a manner that is direct and straightforward. Page 9.

body burden(s): the quantity of a particular chemical from the external environment stored in the body tissues at any given time, especially a toxin to which the body is exposed. The types of body burdens that can exist in the tissues include drugs, toxic chemicals and radioactive substances. Page 166.

body-soluble: capable of being melted or dissolved by the body. Page 108.

bomb testing: any of the programs of exploding nuclear bombs in tests that started in 1945 and continued for many years following. Page 169.

B$_1$: a vitamin found in green peas, beans, egg yolks, liver and the outer coating of cereal grains. It assists in the absorption of carbohydrates and enables carbohydrates to release the energy required for cellular function. A *carbohydrate* is one of the three main classes of food (the others are fats and protein) that provide energy to the body. Page 11.

borne out: proven to be true; confirmed. Page 21.

bounce back: recover strength, spirits, good humor, etc., quickly, as after an illness, setback or problem. Page 152.

break (broken) down: make a substance separate into parts or change into another form in a chemical process. Page 20.

breakdown: a failure to operate or an interruption of the operation of (a society or culture); a collapse. Page 10.

brief, in: used to introduce a summary. Page 2.

bringing to light: revealing or making known. Page 12.

bronchial: relating to or affecting the tubes (bronchi) that carry air from the windpipe into the lungs. Inflammation of the bronchial tubes is known as *bronchitis*. Page 70.

bugged: annoyed or bothered. Page 146.

building block: literally, a large block of concrete or similar hard material used for building houses and other large structures. Hence anything thought of as a basic unit of construction regarded as contributing to something's growth or development. Page 7.

burn-out: of or relating to the point when a person in contact with radioactive materials would be likely to absorb more radiation than the body could tolerate, leading to becoming ill from radiation sickness. *See also* **radiation sickness.** Page 170.

burnt sienna: a paint that has a reddish-brown color. The name comes from a type of earth that is used for coloring paint, originally from Siena, Italy, and which is heated in a furnace to achieve the rust color. Page 158.

burn-up: the action of using up completely; exhausting the supply of. Page 45.

burn up: use up completely; exhaust the supply of. Page 46.

by far: to the most extreme or evident degree. Page 80.

C: a water-soluble vitamin found in citrus fruits, tomatoes, raw onions, raw potatoes and leafy green vegetables. It helps promote healthy gums and teeth, aids in mineral absorption, helps heal wounds and aids the prevention and treatment of the common cold. Vitamin C reacts with any foreign substance reaching the blood and helps to detoxify the system and prevent toxic reactions caused by drugs. Page 45.

cadmium: a soft, silvery-white metallic element. It is often mixed with other metals to improve their qualities, as of hardness, etc., and is used in paints and batteries. Cadmium is poisonous, leading to serious illness or death if inhaled. Small amounts of cadmium entering the body over long periods may also damage the kidneys and deform bones. Page 158.

calcium: a mineral the body requires for healthy teeth and bones. It occurs naturally in various foods, including dairy products and dark-green leafy vegetables. Page 48.

calcium gluconate: a form of calcium used to prevent and treat calcium deficiencies and as a mineral supplement. (*Gluconate* is a substance obtained from *glucose,* a type of sugar occurring naturally in fruits, honey and blood.) Page 131.

Cal-Mag: calcium, magnesium and vinegar, combined in the correct quantities, in water. Page 66.

cancer: a serious disease in which cells in a person's body increase rapidly in an uncontrolled way, producing abnormal growths. Page 14.

carbon tetrachloride: a clear, nonflammable, highly toxic liquid that will not mix with water. It is used as a solvent, an insecticide, a refrigerant and in fire extinguishers. Page 156.

case histories: detailed accounts of the facts affecting the development or condition of a person or group under treatment or study. Page 69.

case(s): 1. an instance of something; an occurrence; an example. Page 10.

2. any individuals or matters requiring or undergoing official or formal observation, study, investigation, etc. Page 21.

catalytic: involving or causing an increase in the rate of a chemical reaction by the use of a *catalyst,* a substance that increases the rate of a chemical reaction without itself undergoing any change. Page 55.

cell(s): the smallest structural unit of an organism that is capable of independent functioning. All plants and animals are materially made up of one or more cells (the human body has more than 10 trillion) that usually combine to form various tissues. Page 37.

cellular: relating to or consisting of living cells (the smallest structural unit of an organism). Every second of the day, millions of cells in the human body die and are replaced by new cells as an essential part of the normal cycle of cellular activity. Page 8.

chaos: a state of utter confusion or disorder; a total lack of organization or order. Page 100.

chemical-oriented: directed or related (oriented) to the use of *chemicals,* substances, simple or complex, that are the building blocks of matter. Page 7.

chemicals: substances, simple or complex, that are the building blocks of matter. Page 7.

chemical warfare: military operations involving poisonous gases and chemicals as weapons. Page 9.

chemistry: the branch of science that deals with the identification of the substances of which matter is composed, the investigation of their properties and the ways in which they interact, combine and change and the use of these processes to form new substances. Page 107.

chills: unnaturally lowered body temperature accompanied by shivering. Page 55.

chiropractor: one whose occupation is the practice of *chiropractic,* a system of healing based upon the theory that disease results from a lack of normal nerve function. It employs treatment by manipulation and specific adjustment of body structures (as the spinal column) and uses physical therapy, when necessary, to restore proper alignment. Page 149.

chlorinated: that has been treated with chlorine, especially to kill harmful organisms. *Chlorine* is a poisonous chemical element used in small amounts in many everyday items, such as to kill bacteria in drinking water and prevent algae from growing in swimming pools. It is also used in paper production, disinfectants, food, insecticides, paints, plastics, medicines and many other products. Page 71.

chronic: lasting for a long period of time or marked by frequent recurrence. Page 167.

chronicle: a written record of events in the order in which they happened. Page 2.

cider vinegar: vinegar made from apple *cider,* the juice pressed from apples. *Vinegar* is a sour-tasting liquid used to flavor and preserve foods. Page 132.

circulation: the movement of blood around the body. Page 20.

cited: mentioned as an example to support an argument or help explain what is being said. Page 103.

civilization: all the people in the world and the societies they live in, considered as a whole. Also, any society, with its culture and its way of life, at a particular period of time or in a particular part of the world. Page 2.

Civil Service Technical Guild: an organization of New York City employees with technical training (such as engineers, architects, scientists and the like) who are responsible to design and maintain the city's bridges, highways, subways, etc. A *guild* is an association of people for mutual aid. *Civil service* means those who work for the government of a city, state, country, etc., not including the military and judicial branches and elected politicians. Page 165.

claim(s): a statement that something is a fact. Page i.

clammy: unpleasantly moist, cold and sticky. Page 41.

clamping down: *clamp* means hold something tightly. *Clamping down* means taking strict action to prevent something. Page 41.

clean up: eradicate harmful influences or elements (from within something). Page 28.

clinical: of, relating to or connected with a clinic (a facility devoted to the diagnosis and care of patients who receive treatment without staying overnight). Page 22.

coal tar: a thick, black, sticky liquid produced in the processing of coal. Coal tar compounds are used in making dyes, drugs, explosives, food flavorings, perfumes, etc. Page 14.

cocaine: a powerful and highly addictive stimulant drug that acts on the central nervous system (the brain and the spinal cord), increasing heart rate and blood pressure while reducing fatigue. Because cocaine can cause dangerous side effects and addiction, it is illegal in many countries. Page 7.

cocktail: any (unpleasant or dangerous) mixture of substances or factors. Page 149.

codeine: a drug obtained from opium, used as a painkiller or sedative and to inhibit coughing. (*Opium* is an addictive drug prepared from the juice of the poppy plant.) Page 22.

cold-pressed: a term used to describe oil that has been extracted from seeds, etc., by pressure alone and without the aid of heat.

In oil extraction, heat is sometimes applied to the seeds to make the oil flow faster, thus increasing the speed of the process; however, the heat may destroy some of the nutritional value of the oil. Page 138.

colitis: inflammation of the colon, characterized by diarrhea, fever, lower-bowel spasms and upper-abdominal cramps. Page 55.

commonplace: encountered often. Page 8.

compensate: make up (for); be equivalent to. Page 42.

composite: 1. something made of different parts or elements. Page 47. **2.** of or having to do with something made of different parts or elements. Page 99.

compositions: materials or substances prepared from or composed of various ingredients. Page 107.

compound(s): 1. a substance composed of two or more parts in exact proportions. Page 8.
2. increase or intensify. Page 15.

comprehend: grasp mentally; understand. Page 99.

comprehensive: including everything, so as to be complete. Page 24.

compulsion: a powerful or irresistible force or drive to do something or take a particular course of action. Page 108.

concern: worry or anxiety that comes from an interest in (someone or something). Page 1.

concurred: had the same opinion or reached agreement on a specified point; agreed. Page 160.

conditioning: causing to become accustomed to something, making someone or something adapt (to a particular situation, treatment, environment, etc.). Page 55.

conductivity: the ability to transmit electric impulses; the allowing of electrical impulses to travel along something such as a wire, nerve channel, etc. Page 108.

conjunction with, in: together with. *Conjunction* means an instance of coming together. Page 54.

construed: interpreted or understood in a particular way, often apart from the way something really is. Page i.

consumption: the eating or drinking (of something) or the amount that a person eats or drinks. Page 12.

contractor: an individual with a formal contract to do a specific job, supplying labor and materials or providing and overseeing staff, if needed, especially those who do so in any of the building trades. Page 157.

contrary, to the: to the opposite effect; in reversal of what is stated. Page 96.

contributive: 1. tending to give something that helps to achieve a specific purpose. Page 45.

2. tending to be one of the causes of something. Page 47.

convulsion(s): violent shakings of the body or limbs caused by uncontrollable muscle contractions. Page 115.

cope: face and deal with responsibilities, problems or difficulties, especially successfully or in an adequate manner. Page 80.

copper: a trace (very small amount) element that is essential in nutrition and needed to absorb and utilize iron. Copper is used in healing and in the production of energy and healthy nerves and joints. Deficiency signs (which are rare) include weakness, impaired breathing and growth, and poor use of iron. Page 126.

count: a reference to a measurement of radiation as measured on a Geiger counter (an instrument that is used for detecting and measuring radioactivity). If something has a high count, it is highly radioactive. Page 15.

counteract: prevent something having an effect or lessen its effect. Page 116.

course of, in the: during the progress or length of. Page 53.

course, run (its): proceed through a regular series of stages. Said of a sensation, manifestation or the like that gradually becomes less and less until it finally disappears. Page 69.

cross-reaction: a (sometimes negative) response that comes from both sides of something. *Cross* in this sense means involving a mutual interchange. Page 27.

crystal(s): small, irregular solid formations of material, used here specifically referring to small deposits of LSD (or any similar drug) stored in the tissues of the body. Page 25.

culture: the pattern (if any) of life in the society. All factors of the society—social, educational, economic, etc., whether creative or destructive. Page 10.

cumulative: increasing in effect, size, quantity, etc., by successive additions. Page 15.

damned: used to express amazement. Page 168.

data: facts or information, especially when examined and used to find out things or make decisions. Page i.

debilitated: weakened or reduced in strength or energy. Page 10.

deduce: derive as a conclusion from something already known or assumed. Page 103.

deduction: something that is deduced. *See also* **deduce.** Page 103.

defeatist mechanism: a means of causing people to surrender easily or no longer resist defeat because of the conviction that further effort is futile (incapable of producing any result). Page 9.

defend: protect (something) from attack, harm or danger. Page 49.

deficiency(ies): the state of not having, or not having enough of, something that is essential. Page 45.

defined: clearly outlined or characterized. Page 70.

dehydrated: lacking water in the body, as the result of loss of bodily fluids or from being deprived of liquid. Page 40.

delirium tremens (D.T.'s): a condition caused by excessive and prolonged use of alcoholic liquors and characterized by hallucinations, mental confusion, restlessness, sweating and trembling. Page 46.

delusive: characterized by *delusion,* a fixed false belief; something that is perceived in a way different from the way it is in reality. From the word *delude,* which means to mislead the mind or judgment of, and *illusion,* which means something that deceives by producing a false or misleading impression of reality. Page 108.

depletion: a reduction of something by a large amount so that there is not enough left. Page 40.

deposit(s): an accumulation of material in a body tissue, structure or fluid. Page 21.

depressant: also called *sedative,* a drug or agent that has the effect of slowing the rate of the body's muscular or nervous activity. Page 12.

depression: a feeling of sadness in which a person feels there is no hope for the future. Page 169.

derivative: a substance obtained from, or regarded as having come from, another substance. Page 14.

derived: acquired or drawn (from something). Page 107.

despair: complete loss of hope regarding some thing or action; feelings of defeat. Page 100.

detonation(s): a violent explosion, as of a bomb. Page 168.

detoxification: the action of removing a poison or a poisonous effect from something, such as from one's body. Page 8.

devastating: causing enormous shock, upset or destruction. Page 11.

devastation: great destruction or damage, especially over a wide area. Page 2.

deviation: departure from a standard or normal procedure. Page 80.

dexterity: skill in using the hands or body; also, mental skill or cleverness. Page 96.

diagnosis: the process of determining the nature and circumstances of an illness or disorder. This is done by means of interview, physical examination, medical tests and other procedures. Also, the decision reached from such an examination. Page 160.

Dianetics: *Dianetics* means "through the mind" or "through the soul" (from Greek *dia,* through, and *nous,* mind or soul). It is a system of coordinated axioms which resolve problems concerning human behavior and psychosomatic illnesses. It combines a workable technique and a thoroughly validated method for increasing sanity, by erasing unwanted sensations and unpleasant emotions.

diesel: involved with or relating to a type of heavy-duty engine (diesel engine) used in some cars but mainly trucks. The diesel engine was invented by German engineer and inventor Rudolf Diesel (1858–1913). Page 155.

diet: 1. used to describe a food or drink that is intended for people trying to lose weight, usually because it is low in calories or fat or contains a sugar substitute. Page 13.

2. the food that a person eats and drinks regularly. Page 23.

dietary: relating to what people eat. Page 45.

dioxin: a highly toxic chemical that occurs in some pesticides and defoliants (chemicals that remove leaves from trees), known to cause cancer and birth defects. Page 13.

disarrange: unsettle or disturb the order or proper arrangement of; throw out of order. Page 22.

discharge: go away so as to be free or rid of (something). Page 56.

disciplinary: relating to the enforcing of rules and the punishing of people who break them. Page 104.

dislodge: force or knock something out of its position. Page 21.

dispelled: caused to be removed. Page 21.

dissipate: diminish; fade or vanish. Page 71.

distorted: changed in shape or appearance so that (something) is not clear or in the correct order. Page 24.

dominant: more important, powerful or noticeable (than other things). Page 19.

do people in: attack or kill people. Page 12.

dormant: temporarily inactive or not in use. Page 34.

dosage(s): an amount of something, usually a vitamin, medicine or drug, that is taken regularly over a particular period of time. Page i.

dramatic: great, marked or strong, etc. Page 53.

dramatization: a repeating in action of what has happened to one in experience. More importantly, it is a replay now of something that happened then, out of its time and period. Page 108.

druggies: drug addicts. Page 10.

Drug Rundown: done after the Purification Program, this rundown unburdens the effects of a person's drug use. By addressing the mental and spiritual damage that results from drug use, one experiences considerable relief and expansion as a spiritual being. The result is a person released from the mental and spiritual effects of drugs, medicine and alcohol. *See also* **rundown.** Page 19.

drum: a large cylindrical container used for storing liquids, for example, oil or chemicals. Page 14.

dry heaves: the action of making sounds and movements as if one is vomiting but without actually doing so. Page 169.

ease: 1. make something less unpleasant, painful, severe, etc. Page 116. **2.** freedom from difficulty or great effort. Page 159.

educated: as if in possession of intellectual powers. Page 51.

effect: bring about; accomplish; make happen. Page 96.

efficacy: capability of producing a desired result or effect; effectiveness. Page 50.

elemental: consisting of a single chemical element (one of a class of substances that cannot be separated into simpler substances by chemical means) in uncombined form. Page 131.

element(s): anything, whether material or immaterial, that forms a part of a whole. Page 8.

eliminated: removed or gotten rid of. Page 22.

elimination, processes of: procedures for the removal of something. Used here in reference to the usual routes (such as the pores of the skin) by which a body gets rid of unwanted particles from within it. Page 21.

embarked upon: began (a new project or course of action). Page 2.

embedded: firmly or deeply fixed in a surrounding mass. Page 22.

emitted: sent out, said of something such as odor, light, heat, sound, gas, etc. Page 71.

empirical: based on scientific testing or practical experience, not on ideas or theory. Page 103.

employed: made use of. Page 103.

end-all in itself: a purpose or goal desired for its own sake (rather than to attain something else). Page 28.

endocrine: of or produced by the *endocrine system,* a system of glands that help the nervous system regulate various body activities, including growth, development and reproduction as well as proper chemical composition of the blood and the body's responses to stress. Page 48.

End Phenomena: indicators which are present when an action has been fully and correctly completed. *Phenomena* is plural of *phenomenon,* an observable fact or event. Page 85.

English system: a reference to the units of measurement used in the United States (ounces, pounds, yards, etc.). This system was brought over from England by the early settlers and has remained the standard of measurement. Page 133.

"enhancer(s)": something designed to improve, but which actually reduces, the quality of something. Page 13.

erratically: in a manner that is not even or regular in pattern or movement; unpredictably. Page 79.

essential: necessary; important in a particular situation or for a particular activity. Page 15.

essential fatty acids: *fatty acids* are the key building blocks of all fats and oils, both in food and in the body. They are the main components of the fat stored in fat cells, which serve as important sources of stored energy, are the main component of the membranes that surround all cells and play key roles in the construction and maintenance of all healthy cells. *Essential fatty acids* are those that the body does not make, but which must be gotten from food. Page 61.

essentially: basically or fundamentally, used when referring to the true or basic nature of something. Page 9.

etherlike: resembling or similar to *ether,* a colorless liquid with a pleasant smell. It is used as a solvent and was formerly used as an anesthetic. Page 71.

ethical: of or having to do with agreed principles of correct moral conduct. Page 11.

evening primrose: a plant with hairy leaves and yellow flowers that open in the evening, whose seeds yield an oil having uses as a food supplement. Page 141.

evidence: show or indicate by a particular action or occurrence. Page 141.

evidently: clearly. Used to indicate that something is undoubtedly true because it is there to be seen. Page 28.

evolved: worked out or developed especially by experience, experimentation or intensive care or effort. Page 21.

exceeding: going beyond the bounds or limits (of something) in quantity, degree or scope. Page 2.

excess(ive): more than is necessary, reasonable or acceptable. Page 15.

exchange: hand something over and receive as a replacement something more suitable or more satisfactory. Used figuratively. Page 59.

exclusively: solely and only; limited to one thing and excluding everything else. Page 59.

expelling: a forcing of something out of the body or out of a part of the body. Page 41.

expose: cause someone to experience or be at risk of. Page 12.

exposure: the experience of coming into contact with something, such as an environmental condition, that has a harmful effect. Page 14.

extensive: 1. very complete, thorough or far-reaching. Page 2.
2. great in amount or number. Page 15.

extract: a substance that has been taken out of a compound by using an industrial or chemical process. Page 14.

extremities: the parts of the body that are furthest from the center, especially the hands and feet. Page 71.

extroverted: having one's interest and attention outward or to things outside oneself. Page 147.

exudation: the giving off or oozing out (of moisture), in the manner of sweat through the pores. Page 21.

eyes, in (one's): in one's own opinion, estimation or judgment; from one's own point of view. Page 151.

face of, in the: when confronted with; in the presence of. Page 49.

factor(s): a circumstance, fact or influence that contributes to a condition, situation or result. Page 1.

faddism: a fondness for fads or a tendency to follow fads. A *fad* is a temporary fashion, idea, manner of conduct, etc., that is embraced with great enthusiasm and that is usually short-lived. Page 9.

fallacy: a deceptive, misleading or false idea, belief, etc. Page 95.

fallout: airborne radioactive dust and material shot into the atmosphere by a nuclear explosion, which then settles to the ground. Page 15.

fashion: a particular way of doing something. Page 72.

fatigue: extreme tiredness. Page 158.

fat(s): one of the three main classes of food (the others are proteins and carbohydrates) that provide energy to the body. Fats provide a highly concentrated source of energy for the cells; serve as building blocks for the membranes that surround every cell in the body; and help blood to clot and the body to absorb certain vitamins. Fats occur in foods derived from both animals and vegetables. Page 20.

fatty acids, (essential): *fatty acids* are the key building blocks of all fats and oils, both in food and in the body. They are the main components of the fat stored in fat cells, which serve as important sources of stored energy, are the main component of the membranes that surround all cells and play key roles in the construction and maintenance of all healthy cells. *Essential fatty acids* are those that the body does not make, but which must be gotten from food. Page 61.

fatty tissue: a kind of body tissue containing stored fat that serves as a source of energy; it also cushions and insulates vital organs. Page 20.

fiber: 1. an essential character or quality. Page 11.

2. the coarse, fibrous substances in grains, fruits and vegetables that normally pass undigested through the body. Eating fiber is said to aid digestion and help to clean out the intestines. Page 49.

film: literally, a thin layer covering a surface. Used figuratively to refer to something acting like a thin cover that causes one's vision to be blurry. Page 152.

first responder: a public safety officer (such as a firefighter, police officer or emergency medical technician) who arrives first at the scene of a disaster, accident or other emergency and who provides immediate assistance and medical aid. Page 163.

fission: the splitting (fissioning) of the nucleus (center) of an atom into fragments, accompanied by a tremendous release of energy. Page 15.

flanked: strengthened or protected. From *flank,* the extreme right or left side of an army or fleet; thus to *flank* means to defend or guard at the flank. Page 117.

flare up: (of an illness) suddenly start again. Page 70.

flashback(s): a memory, past incident or event occurring again vividly in one's mind. Specifically, with certain drugs (such as LSD and similar drugs), it is the reemergence of some aspect of the hallucination (which took place while on the drug) in the absence of taking the drug. The most common form includes altered visual images; wavering, altered borders to visual images; or trails of light. Page 21.

flush: a red color that appears on the face or body, sometimes when hot, or the hot feeling itself, within the body. Page 54.

flush (out): get rid of harmful substances in a part of the body or the whole body by using a large amount of liquid. Page 21.

fly off: a shortened form of *fly off the handle,* to lose one's temper, especially without justification. Page 153.

fog, in a: in a state of mental confusion or unawareness. Page 147.

fog, out of the: out of a state of mental confusion or unawareness. Page 153.

foodstuff(s): a substance that can be eaten, especially one of the basic elements of the human diet. Page 48.

formula: 1. a recipe or prescription giving method and proportions of ingredients for the preparation of some material (such as a combination of vitamins, a medicine or the like). Page 66.
2. a set form of words, a description, statement or the like, as for indicating a procedure to be followed, an expression of a principle, etc. Page 109.

frustrated: annoyed or impatient (with something or someone). Page 148.

full-blown: possessing all the qualities or features to be fully or completely developed. Page 40.

fully: entirely or wholly; to the full extent of the time, quantity or number specified. Page 15.

fumes: gas that has a strong, unpleasant odor and that is dangerous to breathe. Page 156.

gain: an improvement or resurgence; any betterment of the individual. Page 27.

gallstones: small hard masses that form in the gallbladder, sometimes as a result of infection or blockage. The *gallbladder* is a small baglike bodily organ connected to the liver that stores a liquid that helps the body digest food, especially fats. Page 141.

gastroenteritis: inflammation of the stomach and intestines, causing vomiting and diarrhea. *Gastro* means stomach. *Entero* means intestines and *-itis* means inflammation or swelling. Page 55.

generate: produce or create something. Page 37.

generation: a single stage in the descent of a family or a group of people, or the individuals belonging to the same stage. Page 104.

get the best of: defeat somebody in some way or be more than somebody can control. Page 153.

ghastly: extremely unpleasant or bad; terrible. Page 115.

glandular: of or relating to the glands. A *gland* is a mass of cells or an organ in the body that produces particular chemical substances for use in the body. For example, adrenal glands produce adrenaline, a substance that is released into the bloodstream in response to physical or mental stress, as from fear of injury. It initiates many bodily responses, including stimulation of heart action and increase in blood pressure. Page 48.

gm: an abbreviation for *gram,* which is equal to 0.035 ounce. Page 125.

goes without saying: is completely self-evident; is understood. Page 34.

goofy: silly or stupid. Page 147.

grade, poor-: being of a quality rated as low or inferior. Page 132.

gradient(ly): a gradual approach to something, taken step by step, level by level, each step or level itself easily attainable. Page 23.

graduated: divided into or arranged in regular or proportional steps, grades or intervals. Page 72.

grain(s): the smallest unit of weight in the system of weights used in the United States, Great Britain and Canada, originally based on the weight of a single grain of wheat. A grain weighs 1/7,000 pound and is equal to approximately 0.065 gram. Page 10.

gristly: having a texture resembling that of gristle in toughness, etc. (*Gristle* is a tough connective tissue found in humans that provides support to the skeleton at specific sites throughout the body, such as in the nose, throat and ears.) Page 59.

Ground Zero: the site of the World Trade Center attacks on 11 September 2001. Originally a term referring to that part of the ground situated immediately under an exploding nuclear weapon. Page 163.

grudgingly: as if in a reluctant or unwilling manner. Page 169.

Gulf War Syndrome, (Persian): a collective group of medical ailments reported by veterans who served in the 1991 Persian Gulf War. The term *Gulf War Syndrome* or *Illness* emerged in the years following the war, when up to 100,000 of the 697,000 United States troops who had served in the Persian Gulf came to Veterans Affairs Medical Centers with complaints of mysterious ailments they attributed to their wartime service. Research has shown that the syndrome is a consequence of exposure to a variety of substances, including pesticides and chemical and biological warfare agents as well as substances used to counteract poisonous chemicals. Page 166.

habitually: by habit; in a way that is constantly repeated or continued. Page 96.

hallucination: the perception of objects with no reality and the experiencing of sensations without any external cause; the apparent perception (usually by sight or hearing) of an external object when no such object is actually present. The condition is brought about by drugs or severe illness. Page 25.

hanging up: getting stuck so as to remain or persist. Page 73.

harboring: keeping or holding in the mind; maintaining. Page 10.

hard: 1. highly addictive and particularly dangerous to the health. Page 70.

2. to an extreme degree. Page 73.

harder: 1. more difficult and involving an even greater amount of effort or persistence. Page 95.

2. with more effort or force; more thoroughly. Page 104.

hard put, be: have considerable difficulty or trouble. Page 7.

hashish: a drug formed from the flowering tops of the hemp plant. It is smoked or chewed for its narcotic ("pain reducing" or "relaxing") properties. It markedly alters thinking, judgment and complex coordination such as that needed to drive a car. Page 70.

headlines, make the: be an important item of news in newspapers or on the radio or television. A *headline* is the title of a newspaper article printed in large letters, especially at the top of the front page. Page 100.

heat exhaustion: a condition characterized by faintness, rapid pulse, nausea and cool skin, caused by loss of adequate fluid and salt from the body and prolonged exposure to heat. Page 40.

heatstroke: a disturbance of the temperature-regulating mechanisms of the body caused by overexposure to excessive heat, resulting in fever, hot and dry skin, and rapid pulse. Page 41.

heavy: (of a person) using or consuming something a great deal. Page 12.

heroin: a compound derived from morphine (a drug used in medicine to relieve pain) that is illegally used as a powerful and addictive drug causing a lessened sensation of pain, slowed breathing and depression. Withdrawal symptoms include cramplike pains in the limbs, sweating, anxiety, chills, severe muscle and bone aches, fever and more. If overdosed, it can be fatal. Page 10.

high blood pressure: abnormally high pressure of the blood against the inner walls of the blood vessels. Page 34.

hit upon: reached or found. Page 46.

hives: a skin rash that is marked by itching and small pale or red swellings and often lasts for a few days. Page 55.

hold true: be, or continue to be, true; prove true or applicable over time. *Hold* is used here to mean maintain a condition, situation, course of action, etc., over time. Page 10.

host: a very large number; a great quantity. Page 21.

hostilities: unfriendly or aggressive feelings or behavior. Page 10.

hung over: of or concerning a headache and sick feeling as a result of drinking too much alcohol. Page 71.

hung up: halted or snagged. Page 26.

hypnotics: drugs or other agents that cause sleep or drowsiness. Page 107.

illicit: not allowed by the law; not approved of by the normal rules of a society. Page 19.

ills: problems, difficulties or things considered harmful. Page 11.

impede: interfere with the movement, progress or development of something. Page 8.

improbable: not likely to happen. Page 168.

impulse: a sudden urge that prompts an act or feeling. Page 95.

impurities: substances that are added to something else so that it is no longer pure. Impurities in the body can include drugs and other toxic chemical substances—for example, food preservatives, insecticides, pesticides, as well as any residual crystals of drugs (if the person has ever taken LSD or any similar drug). Page 37.

in: things which should be there and are or should be done and are, are said to be "in." For example, *"points that must be in on a Purification Program."* Page 42.

in a fog: in a state of mental confusion or unawareness. Page 147.

in brief: used to introduce a summary. Page 2.

incalculable: too great to be measured. Page 56.

incident(s): an experience, simple or complex, related by the same subject, location or people, understood to take place in a short and finite time period such as minutes or hours or days. Page 19.

indebted: grateful to somebody for something such as assistance or a favor received. Page 59.

indeed: used to give additional emphasis to a descriptive word or phrase. Page 103.

in-depth: very thorough and detailed. Page 24.

indicator(s): a sign or symptom that gives evidence of or shows (something). Page 22.

induced: brought about, produced or caused by. Page 25.

industrial: relating to or involving companies that manufacture or sell a particular product or range of products that are made from raw materials, as opposed to products that are grown and then sold. Page 9.

infinity: a large amount that is impossible to count. Page 100.

ingest: take something (such as food, a liquid or a gas) into the body by swallowing, inhaling or absorbing it. Page 14.

inhalers: small devices used for inhaling medicine in the form of a vapor or gas in order to ease a breathing condition. Page 154.

in light of: taking into consideration what is known, or what has just been said or found out. Page 15.

in short: introducing a summary statement of what has been previously stated in a few words; in summary. Page 9.

insidious: (of something dangerous) gradually and secretly causing harm. Page 146.

in spite of: regardless of; without being affected by the particular factor mentioned. Page 96.

instigator: a person who gets something started. Page 45.

insulation: protective material that prevents heat from passing through. Page 38.

intake: an amount taken in (by the body) or the act of taking something into the body, usually by swallowing or inhaling something. Page 7.

in tandem: in association or partnership. Page 66.

integral: being an essential part of something; necessary to the completeness of the whole. Page 54.

intensity: the strength, power, force or concentration of something. Page 38.

interaction: the action or influence of persons or things on each other. Page 7.

interfere with (something): prevent (something) from happening as planned or as part of its usual course of action. Page 8.

intestinal walls: the *intestine* is a long tube in the body between the stomach and the anus that digests and absorbs food. *Intestinal walls* refers to the sides of the intestinal tube. Page 66.

in the course of: during the progress or length of. Page 53.

in the face of: when confronted with; in the presence of. Page 49.

intoxication: drunkenness; a state of being affected with lessened physical and mental control by means of alcoholic liquor, a drug or another substance. Page 71.

in utero: a Latin phrase meaning in or while still inside a woman's uterus; unborn. Page 34.

in view of (something): because of (something). Used to introduce the reason for a decision, action or situation. Page 28.

iodine: a mineral which is required in trace (very small) amounts for normal growth, extracted from brine (very salty water) or from certain seaweeds called *kelp* which contain especially high concentrations of iodine. Page 126.

ion: an electrically charged atom or group of atoms. An atom becomes an ion if it loses or gains an electron (any of the negatively charged particles that form a part of all atoms). Atoms of different elements do not always join together, but their ions might. Ions can join together to form new substances that are held together by the electric charge. Page 66.

iron: a mineral that is essential to the body's healthy function. Most of the iron in the body is found in the red blood cells where it is needed to help the transfer of oxygen between the blood and the rest of the body. The first signs of iron deficiency are a washed-out feeling, weakness, fatigue and a decreased ability for physical activity. Page 126.

iron men and wooden ships: a reference to the early navies whose wooden-hulled vessels with sail power required sailors with physical strength and an "iron" will. Page 108.

IU: abbreviation for *International Unit,* a measured unit based on an internationally standard amount of something (such as a vitamin) needed to bring about a certain response in the body. Page 125.

jellyfish: a marine animal, characteristically having a semisolid, umbrellalike body and long poisonous tentacles for stinging. Some types of jellyfish found in the southern parts of the Pacific

Ocean, such as in areas off the coasts of Australia, are known to be among the most poisonous animals on Earth. Page 159.

junk foods: foods that do not form part of a well-balanced diet, especially highly processed, high-fat snack items eaten in place of or in addition to regular meals. Page 49.

keeling over: falling over or collapsing suddenly, as if from fainting. Page 38.

kick: a strong but temporary interest or activity. Page 9.

kicks: thrill or excitement. Page 95.

kidney(s): of or pertaining to the *kidneys,* a pair of organs in the lower back whose functions include removing waste products from the blood in the form of urine and regulating the amount of fluid in the body. Page 34.

kiloton(s): a measure of force used with reference to the explosive capability of a nuclear weapon. One kiloton is equivalent to the explosion of a thousand tons of *TNT,* a chemical substance that is a powerful explosive. Page 168.

lamentable: bad; unfortunate; distressing. Page 109.

large, at: as a whole; in general; (taken) altogether. Page 9.

lasting: continuing or remaining for a long time; permanent. Page 1.

lecithin: a waxy substance that is important in human cell function and that occurs especially in nerve tissue and red blood cells. Commercial forms of lecithin, which are produced mainly from egg yolks and from soybean oil, are used in a variety of foods and medicines. Page 61.

letdown: a decline or decrease in spirit or energy, especially after a feeling of well-being. Page 127.

lethargic: lacking energy, activity or enthusiasm. Page 147.

level off: become (more) stable. Page 148.

licensed medical practitioner: a person licensed to practice medicine; a medical doctor; physician. Page 33.

life-hostile: that makes life difficult. *Hostile* here means situations and conditions that make it difficult to achieve something (such as living). Page 8.

light, bringing to: revealing or making known. Page 12.

line of duty: all that is authorized, required or normally associated with a field of responsibility, such as of a soldier, police officer, firefighter, etc. Page 166.

linseed: a yellowish oil used, because of its drying qualities, in making paints and printing inks, for protecting wood surfaces, etc. Page 157.

litany: a long and often repeated list (of something, such as complaints, problems, etc.). Page 10.

lithium: a chemical element used by psychiatry since the late 1940s as a supposed treatment for manic depression. Some of the side effects from its use are nausea, stomach cramps, diarrhea, thirstiness, blurred vision, confusion, abnormal muscle movement and pulse irregularities. Page 11.

liver: an organ in the body that stores and filters blood and takes part in many other functions. Page 70.

living proof: evidence that is conclusive, that serves to establish the truth of something and that is alive and real, specifically a person in a specific condition that demonstrates the validity of a statement. Page 169.

lock up: become fixed or immobile; stuck. Page 20.

lodge: become fixed, implanted or caught in a place or position; come to rest; stick. Page 20.

logical: (of an action, event, etc.) seeming natural, reasonable or sensible. Page 16.

long-range: extending into the future. Page 27.

Los Alamos: a town in central New Mexico. It is the location of the *Los Alamos National Laboratory,* the site chosen in 1942 for research and development of nuclear weapons. Page 169.

LSD: a type of *hallucinogen,* a group of drugs that produce psychological problems and often physical damage. It was originally used by psychiatrists to bring about temporary psychotic breaks in patients and became widely used illegally in the 1960s. Mild effects produced by low doses can include feelings of detachment from the surroundings, emotional swings and an altered sense of space and time. With higher doses, visual disturbances and illusions occur. Large dosages can be fatal. *LSD* is an abbreviation for the chemical compound *l(y)s(ergic acid) d(iethylamide).* Page 7.

lukewarm: just slightly warm; moderately warm. Page 42.

magnesium: a mineral that occurs in green leafy vegetables, nuts, peas, beans, etc. Magnesium aids in the proper functioning of nerves and muscles (especially the heart), the body's utilization of fats and in sleeping well. Page 65.

magnesium carbonate: a form of magnesium found naturally in the earth and used in medicines for its calming effect on the nerves. It dissolves in acid but not in water or alcohol. Page 131.

magnitude: quantity or greatness of size, extent, etc. Page 13.

majority: the greater number or part; a number more than half of the total. Page 7.

Man: the human race or species, humankind, Mankind. Page 1.

mandatory: needing to be done, followed or complied with. Page 23.

manganese: a mineral contained in foods such as beans, nuts, green leafy vegetables and cereals that plays a role in increasing fertility and assisting in proper body growth and maintenance of the central nervous system. Page 126.

manifestation(s): a visible demonstration or display of the existence, presence, qualities or nature of something. Page 22.

manikin: a life-size model of the human body. Manikins, automobiles, houses and other structures were used at the Nevada Test Site to show the effects of radiation and blast waves. They were placed at distances from the point where the nuclear bomb was to be exploded and were sometimes photographed from protected locations during the explosion. *See also* **blast** and **Nevada.** Page 168.

manner of, all: many different kinds of; all sorts of. Page 100.

marijuana: a drug made from the dried leaves and flowering tops of the hemp plant. People smoke, chew or eat marijuana. It has effects of intoxication (being affected with lessened physical and mental control) and distortions of sensory perceptions. Marijuana gained widespread use in the United States in the 1960s and 1970s, becoming the second-most-used drug after alcohol. Page 7.

markedly: noticeably, to a significant extent. Page 48.

marrow: soft fatty tissue that fills the central cavities (hollow spaces) of bones. Page 117.

massy: characterized by a sensation of mass. Literally, *mass* is a body of matter that forms a whole and that has weight. *Massy* is used figuratively to describe a sensation as of mass or weight around the head. Page 170.

means: an action, object or system by which a result is achieved; a way of achieving or doing something. Page 21.

measure, in no small: to a large extent or degree. Page 70.

measures: procedures; courses of action or plans (to achieve a particular purpose); also, laws or proposed laws. Page 104.

mechanism, defeatist: a means of causing people to surrender easily or no longer resist defeat because of the conviction that further effort is futile (incapable of producing any result). Page 9.

medication: a drug used in medical treatments; a medicine. Page i.

medium: a specific kind of artistic technique or means of expression as determined by the materials used or the creative methods involved. Also, the materials used in a specific artistic technique. Page 157.

menace: someone or something that is a possible source of danger or harm. Page 108.

mental image pictures: three-dimensional color pictures with sound and smell and all other perceptions, plus the conclusions and speculations of the individual. They are mental copies of one's perceptions sometime in the past. Page 24.

mercury: a silver-colored metal that is liquid at room temperature. Mercury is used in many products, such as thermometers. It is extremely poisonous if inhaled. Small amounts taken into the body repeatedly tend to bring about cumulative poisoning, which can lead to death. Page 156.

metabolize: break down food in the body by chemical activity to produce the materials and energy necessary for life. Page 141.

methadone: a powerful synthetic drug used as a substitute drug in the "treatment" of addiction to heroin. Methadone failed as a "solution" to heroin addiction because people instead became addicted to methadone. The drug has been known to cause death and life-threatening side effects in people taking it. It causes slow or shallow breathing and dangerous changes in heartbeat that may not be felt by the individual. It is also abused by many people who obtain it illegally. Page 116.

233

metric system: a system of weights and measures in use in a large number of countries. The basic units are the meter (39.37 inches) for length and the gram (15.432 grains) for mass or weight. Page 133.

mg: an abbreviation for *milligram,* a unit for measuring weight, one thousandth of a gram. Page 125.

milliliter: a unit of volume equal to one thousandth of a liter (1 liter is equal to 34 ounces). Page 133.

mind-altering: causing pronounced changes in mood, perceptions, behavior or thought patterns. Page 11.

mineral(s): a substance naturally occurring in the earth, used for the growth and maintenance of the body structure, maintaining the digestive juices and the fluids that are found in and around cells. Unlike vitamins, minerals are inorganic (not created by living things). Minerals play an important role in many functions of the body, such as calcium (used by the body for healthy bones and teeth), magnesium (needed for proper function of the nervous system) and sodium (regulates the amount of water in the body's cells). Page 23.

minute: extremely small, as in size, amount or degree. Page 21.

misery: great mental or emotional distress; extreme unhappiness. Also, distress or suffering caused by need or poverty. Page 10.

mode: a style, manner or way of acting or of doing something. Page 148.

monitor: keep track of, regulate or control thoroughly (some process or operation). Page 23.

moody: tending to change unpredictably from a cheerful to a bad-tempered *mood,* a state of mind that someone experiences at a particular time. Page 148.

morphine: a powerful addictive drug used in medicine to relieve severe pain. Because of its painkilling properties, it can produce a feeling of indifference to what is going on in the environment. Other side effects that accompany morphine are nausea and vomiting, as well as constipation. It is sold and used illegally and if overdosed, can cause death. Page 24.

motivation: reason for doing something. Page 28.

multifaceted: having many aspects or phases. Page 168.

must: something that is essential; something that one must do. Page 20.

Narconon: Narconon (meaning *no drugs*) is a nonprofit social betterment organization and global network of drug rehabilitation and drug education centers, founded in 1966. Narconon is dedicated to restoring drug-free lives to drug-dependent people through the use of L. Ron Hubbard's drug rehabilitation methods. Page i.

nature: the basic or essential qualities or character (of someone or something). Page 1.

nausea: a feeling in the stomach that accompanies the urge to vomit. Page 25.

negligible: that can or should easily be disregarded; that is so tiny or unimportant or otherwise of so little consequence as to require or deserve little or no attention. Page 133.

nervous system: the network of nerve cells and nerve fibers that conveys sensations to the brain and motor (pertaining to or involving muscular movement) impulses to organs and muscles. Page 65.

neutral: having no effect on something because it is an equal balance of two or more qualities, etc. Page 8.

Nevada: a state in the western United States. In the southeastern corner of the state, approximately 65 miles (105 kilometers) north of Las Vegas, is the *Nevada Test Site,* 1,360 square miles (3,500 square kilometers) of desert where nuclear bomb tests were conducted (1951–1992). Of the more than nine hundred such tests, approximately one hundred occurred in the atmosphere, mainly during the 1950s, with later testing done underground. *See also* **blast.** Page 168.

New Hampshire: a state in the northeastern United States. Page 167.

New Mexico: a state in the southwestern United States, where the first atomic bomb was built and exploded during World War II (1939–1945). The bomb was developed at the Los Alamos National Laboratory and was exploded, on 16 July 1945, at a test site in the desert near Alamogordo, in southern New Mexico. *See also* **Los Alamos.** Page 169.

niacin: one of the B complex vitamins which occurs naturally in foods such as cereal grains, eggs, liver and vegetables, and is used in medicine chiefly for preventing skin diseases. Niacin's role on the Purification Program is fully described in Part Two, Chapter Four, "Niacin, the 'Educated' Vitamin." Page 45.

nonoptimum: not the best possible; not producing the best possible results. Page 47.

Novocain: a brand name for an anesthetic (a drug that nullifies pain) used in medicine and dentistry. Page 22.

nuclear: relating to, using or producing energy through nuclear fission or nuclear fusion. Nuclear *fission* is the splitting of the nucleus (central part) of an atom accompanied by a significant release of energy, as used in an atomic bomb. Nuclear *fusion* is the combining of atoms accompanied by a significant release of energy, as used in a hydrogen bomb. Page 9.

numb: unable to feel, think or react in the normal way. Literally, if a part of one's body is numb, one cannot feel anything in it. Page 95.

nutrient(s): a substance that is needed to keep a living body alive and to help it grow. Nutrients are classified as carbohydrates, proteins, fats, vitamins, minerals and water. Page 8.

nutrition: the process by which living things receive the food necessary for them to grow and be healthy. Page 1.

objective: something that one's efforts or actions are intended to attain or accomplish; purpose; goal; target. Page 38.

objective processes: *objective* means "that can be observed." *Objective processes* are those processes that apply to the physical universe. They extrovert the person's attention. *See also* **process(es).** Page 116.

oblivion: a state of unawareness of what is going on. Page 96.

obsessive: pertaining to or resembling an obsession (the domination of one's thoughts or feelings by a persistent idea, image, desire, etc.). Page 96.

occasioned: brought about or caused. Page 47.

oil(s): a liquid fat obtained from plant seeds, animal fats, mineral deposits and other sources that is thicker than and does not dissolve in water. Oils can dissolve or break down other oils. Therefore oil taken into the body can be used to replace bad fat within the body. Page 13.

omega-3 (-6): two essential fatty acids (ones that are not produced by the body and can only be obtained by food or supplements) that are required for the proper functioning of every cell in the body. Without them the body is not able to protect and repair the cells, produce energy by burning fat and calories, generate heat or perform other vital functions. (These essential fatty acids are named according to how the atoms of carbon, a basic chemical element found in all plants and animals, are connected together in a long chain. *Omega* is the name of the carbon atom at the far end of the chain, named after the last letter of the Greek alphabet. *Omega-3* refers to the *third* carbon atom from the end and *omega-6* refers to the *sixth* carbon atom from the end.) Page 137.

onslaught: an attack; especially a vigorous or destructive assault or attack that overwhelms. Page 2.

on-the-job: while in actual performance of one's work. Page 69.

ooze: soft, thick liquid that flows or passes slowly or in small quantities through the pores of the body. Page 167.

operating rule: a principle that works or is being used. Page 27.

operation: a particular form or kind of activity; action. Page 100.

optimum: most favorable or desirable; best. Page 77.

option(s): a choice that is or can be taken. Page 116.

ordered: having all elements in a neat, well-organized or regular arrangement. Page 23.

organic: relating to or derived from living plants and animals. Page 61.

organism: any living thing, such as a human body, plant, animal or bacteria. Page 8.

oriented: directed or related to or toward. Page 7.

outlook: a person's point of view or attitude to life. Page 146.

out of the fog: out of a state of mental confusion or unawareness. Page 153.

outset: the beginning or initial stage of an activity. Page 163.

over-the-counter: directly to a customer, without requiring a doctor's prescription. Page 70.

overused: (of a word or phrase) stated too much or too often, and thereby wearing it out and causing it to have less impact or to lose its full meaning. Page 49.

overwhelmed: affected strongly and made to feel confused or overpowered. Page 25.

palpitations: an irregular or unusually rapid beating of the heart, either because of a medical condition or because of exertion, fear or anxiety. Page 154.

panacea: an answer or solution for all difficulties; cure-all. Page 11.

paraphrase: express the meaning of (something) using different words, especially to achieve greater clarity. Page 108.

partially: not completely or wholly. Page 99.

perceive: notice or become aware of or identify by means of the senses. Page 24.

perceptions: impressions of the environment that enter through the "sense channels," such as the eyes, nose and ears. There are more than fifty perceptions used by the physical body, the best known of which are sight, hearing, touch, taste and smell. Page 24.

period(s): a particular length of time; an interval of time. Page 12.

permeated: spread throughout; affected in every part. Page 8.

per se: a Latin phrase meaning "by itself," used to show that one is referring to something on its own, rather than in connection with other things. Page 15.

Persian Gulf Syndrome: another name for *Gulf War Syndrome,* a collective group of medical ailments reported by veterans who served in the 1991 Persian Gulf War. The term *Gulf War Syndrome* or *Illness* emerged in the years following the war, when up to 100,000 of the 697,000 United States troops who had served in the Persian Gulf came to Veterans Affairs Medical Centers with complaints of mysterious ailments they attributed to their wartime service. Research has shown that the syndrome is a consequence of exposure to a variety of substances, including pesticides and chemical and biological warfare agents as well as substances used to counteract poisonous chemicals. Page 167.

personality: the sum total of the physical, mental, emotional and social characteristics of an individual. Page 10.

perspiration: salty, watery fluid lost from the body by the sweat glands of the skin; sweat. Page 41.

239

pervaded: spread throughout all parts. Page 15.

perverting: changing a system, process, etc., in a bad way so that it is not what it used to be or what it should be. Page 8.

petroleum products: products that are derived from crude oil (petroleum), such as gasoline, natural gas, diesel fuel, heating oil, plastics, paint and synthetic fibers (such as nylon). Page 12.

peyote: a drug made from a small cactus of the same name, native to Mexico and the southwestern United States. Peyote alters perception and can produce hallucinations (a false sense perception of somebody or something that is not really there). Page 24.

pharmaceutical chemicals: chemicals obtained from a pharmacy (a drugstore), as different from illegal drugs. Page 70.

pharmacopeia(s): a book containing an official list of medicinal drugs, together with articles on their preparation and use. Page 54.

phenomenal: extraordinary; highly remarkable. Page 145.

phenomenon: (plural, *phenomena*) an observable fact or event. Page 54.

physiological: of or pertaining to *physiology,* the functions and activities of living organisms and their parts, including all physical and chemical processes. Page 11.

pilot: a preliminary or experimental trial or test serving as a tentative model for future development. Page 2.

pivotal: of vital importance, especially in determining the outcome, progress or success of something. Page 56.

plated: coated with a thin film of gold, silver, etc., as for ornamental purposes. Page 12.

playing against: literally, aiming or directing at, sometimes continuously. Used figuratively. Page 26.

poison(s): any substance that, when introduced into or absorbed by a living body, destroys life or injures health. The term is commonly applied to a substance capable of destroying life by rapid action even when taken in a small quantity. Page 7.

pollutant(s): a substance that is dirty or harmful to the land, air, water, etc., making it no longer pleasant or safe to use. Page 8.

polyunsaturated: belonging to a class of fats, especially plant oils, that are less likely to be converted into cholesterol (an alcohol that, in certain forms, is considered harmful to the heart) in the body. Their molecules have many (poly) carbon atoms that are unsaturated (not bonded or linked up) with hydrogen atoms. Page 138.

poor-grade: being of a quality rated as low or inferior. Page 132.

pore(s): one of the very small holes in the skin that sweat can pass through. Page 38.

pose: present or amount to. Page 9.

pot: a slang name for marijuana. *See also* **marijuana.** Page 147.

potassium: a mineral that occurs in vegetables, fruits, whole grains, nuts and meats and is one of the substances that determines the amount of water held in body tissues. It also attracts nutrients from the intestines into the blood and from the blood into the cells, is essential for muscle contraction and helps in sending messages through the nervous system. Page 40.

potassium gluconate: a chemical compound containing potassium and gluconate (a substance obtained from glucose, a type of sugar occurring naturally in fruits, honey and blood) and is used as a dietary supplement. Page 41.

practitioner, licensed medical: a person licensed to practice medicine; a medical doctor; physician. Page 33.

preaching: urging the acceptance or abandonment of an idea or course of action. Page 49.

precipitation: the factor or factors which cause a sickness to manifest itself. Page 47.

predisposition: a condition which makes one inclined or liable to disease, illness, etc. Page 47.

premise: a proposition that forms the basis of a conclusion. Page 21.

prescribed: 1. (of a drug) directed to be used at set times and in specified amounts. Page 7.

2. laid down as a course of action to be followed. Page 77.

present time: the time which is now and which becomes the past almost as rapidly as it is observed. It is a term loosely applied to the environment existing in now: the ground, sky, walls, objects and people of the immediate environment. In other words, the anatomy of present time is the anatomy of the room or area in which you are at the moment when you view it. Page 24.

preservative: a chemical substance used to keep foods from decaying. Page 7.

"preserver(s)": same as *preservative*. Page 13.

press: the news-gathering business generally or all the people involved in gathering and reporting on the news, but in particular journalists working for newspapers. Page 103.

press for: seek or demand something with urgency. Page 109.

prevalence: the state of being widespread or in general use or acceptance. Page 11.

prevalent: widespread; in general use or acceptance. Page 8.

preventive: undertaken to stop something that causes problems or difficulties from happening. Page 151.

principle(s): a truth, law, doctrine or motivating force upon which something is based. Page 2.

processed: a reference to food that has been treated with chemicals that preserve it or give it extra taste or color. Page 13.

process(es): in Scientology, a precise set of questions asked or directions given to help a person find out things about himself or life and to improve his condition. Page 116.

process(es): a continuous action, operation or series of changes taking place in a definite manner. Page 8.

processes of elimination: procedures for the removal of something. Used here in reference to the usual routes (such as the pores of the skin) by which a body gets rid of unwanted particles from within it. Page 21.

procreate: produce offspring by reproduction. Page 95.

"procreate before death" impulse: a reference to an increased sexual urge that can occur in instances such as starvation, illness, extreme tiredness or the like. Page 95.

proffered: offered for consideration or acceptance. Page 15.

profuse: occurring in large amounts; pouring out freely and abundantly. Page 42.

progressive(ly): by continuous advance; step by step; little by little. Page 45.

prohibit(s): prevent something from occurring. Page 1.

prolonged: lengthened out in time; caused to continue longer. Page 47.

propaganda: information, especially of a biased or misleading nature, used to promote or publicize a particular cause or point of view. Page 96.

proportionate(ly): increasing or decreasing in size, amount or degree in accordance with changes in something else. Page 48.

prospects: the outlook for the future. Page 8.

proven: tested and shown to be true. Page 56.

psychosomatic: *psycho* refers to mind and *somatic* refers to body; the term *psychosomatic* means the mind making the body ill or illnesses which have been created physically within the body by the mind. Page 107.

psychotherapy: the treatment of mental disorders by discussion of an individual's problems, rather than by giving them drugs. Page 116.

publicized: made generally known, typically by advertising. Page 103.

purge: get rid of or remove something undesirable or impure. Page 59.

purportedly: in a way that is claimed or stated but not necessarily proven to be so. Page 141.

pursue: 1. try hard to achieve or obtain something, such as a goal. Page 27.

2. to proceed along, follow or continue with (a specific course, action, plan, etc.). Page 157.

quarters: areas, places, regions or localities. Page 70.

racing: (of the heart) beating much faster than usual as, for example, out of nervousness. Page 25.

radiation: harmful energy sent out from a substance in the form of streams of very small particles due to the decay (breaking down) of atoms within the substance. This energy can be damaging or fatal to the health of people exposed to it. Radiation comes in many forms. The harmful types include atom bomb explosions or, if accumulated in the body, X-rays as used in medicine, and rays from the Sun that cause sunburn. Page 1.

radiation sickness: a medical condition caused by overexposure to radiation as the result of therapeutic treatment, accidental exposure or an atomic bomb explosion. Symptoms include fatigue, headache, vomiting, diarrhea, loss of hair and teeth and, in severe cases, hemorrhaging (uncontrolled bleeding). Page 55.

radically: in a way that departs markedly from the usual or customary; in an extreme manner. Page 116.

radioactive: used to describe a substance that sends out harmful energy in the form of streams of very small particles due to the decay (breaking down) of atoms within the substance. This energy can be damaging or fatal to the health of people exposed to it. Page 8.

rancid: (of oil or of foods containing fat or oil) smelling or tasting unpleasant as a result of being stale. Page 13.

random: having no definite aim or purpose; without pattern or plan. Page 77.

range(s): 1. change or differ within limits. Page 70.
2. the distance which something varies or the limits between which something varies. Page 123.

ran out: past tense of *run out,* be released and eliminated or cause (something) to be released and eliminated. Page 147.

ratio: a number or amount in relationship to another number or amount. For example, if a person spends ten hours inside and one hour outside, the ratio is 10:1, or ten to one. Page 66.

rational: being in full possession of one's reason; sane. Page 11.

rationale: the reasoning or principle that underlies or explains a particular course of action, or a statement setting out these reasons or principles. Page 65.

ration(s): a specified or measured amount of something provided, especially food or drink. Page 48.

ravaging: seriously destructive, damaging or ruinous. Page 19.

raw umber: a paint that has a yellowish-brown color. Page 158.

reaction(s): an instance of responding to something in a particular way or with particular behavior. Page 53.

reactivate: start working or happening again (or be made to start working or happening again) after a period of time has passed. Page 22.

"recreational": not for medical purposes; of or pertaining to a drug that is used occasionally and is claimed to be nonaddictive. Page 70.

rectify: to make, put or set right; remedy; correct. Page 41.

recur: happen or appear once again or repeatedly. Page 54.

regarding: having to do with something; concerning someone or something. Page 9.

regard to, in: concerning someone or something. Used to indicate the subject being talked about. Page 60.

regimen: a specific system, program, plan or course of action to attain some result. Also, a regulated system of diet, exercise, manner of living, etc., intended to preserve or restore health. Page 21.

rehabilitation: a restoring to good condition, health, ability to work, etc. Page i.

reinforced: made stronger by providing additional external support. Page 27.

rejuvenated: restored to a condition characteristic of youthful interest, vigor, enthusiasm, etc. Page 152.

relapse: fall back into an undesirable state or way of life after a period of improvement. Page 19.

release: the act of making something available for the first time or the fact of being made available in this way. Page 2.

rendered: caused to be or become; made. Page 108.

246

replenished: filled again with needed energy or nourishment. Page 40.

reportedly: according to what some people say. Page 10.

representative: typical of something, especially of a class or kind. Page 145.

residual: present or existing, often with the sense of being a quantity left over at the end of an action. Page 13.

residue(s): a small part or quantity that remains after use; remainder. Page 25.

resolution: the action of solving a problem. Page 2.

resounding: very great; impressively complete. Page 2.

respirator(s): a device placed over the nose and mouth to filter out harmful substances so that they are not inhaled. Page 155.

restimulate: reactivate the mental image pictures of a moment of past pain and unconsciousness, triggered by a source unknown to the individual. For example, a person is run into by a truck and then has mental image pictures of pain and unconsciousness. The mental image pictures have a truck in them and are associated with a truck. A few days later the person walks by a similar kind of truck and feels afraid and upset and doesn't know why. What he has done is restimulate the incident of being hit by the truck. The cause of the restimulation is usually unknown to a person. If it were known, the person would immediately recover from it. But if it remains unknown, it tends to be buried and have an effect upon the individual. Page 25.

restimulation: the action or state of being restimulated. *See also* **restimulate.** Page 26.

restimulative: causing restimulation. Page 26.

restore: bring someone or something back to an earlier and better condition. Page 89.

restriction(s): a rule or law that limits what can be done. Page 49.

resurgence: a rising again or springing again into being or vigor. Page 85.

return: that which is given or received, by way of exchange; the outcome of some productive thing. Page 79.

-ridden: full of; burdened with. Page 60.

ridding: freeing the body from something unwanted. Page 21.

riddled: full of; affected with something undesirable that is spread throughout. Page 9.

Ritalin: a type of *amphetamine,* any of a group of powerful stimulant drugs that act on the central nervous system (the brain and the spinal cord), increasing heart rate and blood pressure while reducing fatigue. Ritalin is the most prescribed drug in the world for the supposed psychiatric disorder of "Attention Deficit Hyperactivity Disorder" (ADHD). It is prescribed to adults and children and is highly addictive. Page 11.

root: the basic cause, source or origin of something. Page 103.

round off: make (a figure) less exact but more convenient for calculations, as by increasing or decreasing it to the nearest whole number. Page 133.

Royal Air Force: the British air force, also known by the initials *RAF.* Page 156.

rundown: a series of steps which are processes (drills and exercises) that have specific indicators for completion and are designed to handle a specific aspect of an individual's accumulated upsets, pains, failures, etc. Page 19.

run (its) course: proceed through a regular series of stages. Said of a sensation, manifestation or the like that gradually becomes less and less until it finally disappears. Page 69.

running: operating or functioning; moving forward in time. Page 100.

run out: be released and eliminated or cause (something) to be released and eliminated. Page 55.

safeguard(s): something that is designed to protect from harm, risk or danger. Page 14.

salt substitute: a compound, similar in taste to salt, composed mainly of potassium chloride and consumed chiefly by persons who are supposed to reduce or restrict their intake of sodium chloride (salt) for health reasons. Page 41.

salvage: to rescue or save especially from destruction or ruin. Page 2.

say nothing of: without ever needing to speak of. Used to refer in passing to subjects that might be employed to strengthen what a speaker is saying and has the sense that the speaker is holding back from giving the full strength of his case. Page 108.

schizophrenic(s): a person with two (or more) apparent personalities. *Schizophrenia* means scissors or *two,* plus *head.* Literally, *splitting of the mind,* hence, *split personality.* Page 24.

Scientology: the term *Scientology* is taken from the Latin *scio,* which means "knowing in the fullest sense of the word," and the Greek word *logos,* meaning "study of." In itself the word means literally "knowing how to know." Scientology is further defined as the study and handling of the spirit in relationship to itself, universes and other life.

score, on that: with regard to (the subject under discussion). Page 104.

secondhand smoke: the exhaled smoke and the smoke that floats in the air from cigarettes that are burning. This smoke has been shown to create health problems for those in an environment where secondhand smoke is present. Page 160.

sector: a particular or distinct part (of something). Page 95.

sedative(s): a drug used to bring about sleepiness and temporarily relieve pain and nervousness or agitation. Page 9.

seeping: (of liquids) passing or escaping slowly and in small quantities through an opening or openings, as for example, through the pores of the skin. Page 157.

set off: made (something) start happening. Page 25.

set (someone) up: lead or put into a dangerous or detrimental situation or position. Page 65.

severe: causing discomfort or distress; difficult to endure. Page 25.

sharply: in a manner that is clear and definitely distinct. Page 70.

short, in: introducing a summary statement of what has been previously stated in a few words; in summary. Page 9.

shut-off(s): a temporary interruption or stoppage. Page 96.

side effect(s): 1. an undesirable secondary effect of a drug or other form of medical treatment, such as headaches, weight gain, depression, etc. Page 25.

2. an accompanying result of an action, occurrence or state of affairs. Page 40.

skimp: cut short in time, amount, etc. Page 40.

skip: pass over or leave something out that should properly follow as part of a sequence or a complete work. Page 77.

slight: very small in degree. Page 100.

sodium chloride: common salt as that used to season or preserve food. Page 40.

sole: one and only; unaccompanied by other things or qualities; standing alone. Page 80.

solution: a mixture of two or more substances, such as a solid dissolved in a liquid. Page 66.

solution, into: into the condition of being dissolved. Page 66.

solvent(s): a substance, especially a liquid, that can dissolve other substances. Page 12.

somatic(s): physical pains or discomforts of any kind. It can mean actual pain such as that caused by a cut or a blow. Or it can mean discomfort as from heat or cold. It can mean itching. In short, anything physically uncomfortable. Page 55.

soporifics: drugs or medicines which bring about sleep. Page 107.

spaced out: inattentive, dazed, confused or lightheaded from or as if from drug use. Page 71.

spasms: sudden involuntary contractions, as of muscles, or involuntary movements. Page 65.

speed: slang for *amphetamine,* any of a group of powerful stimulant drugs that act on the central nervous system (the brain and the spinal cord), increasing heart rate and blood pressure while reducing fatigue. Because amphetamines can cause dangerous side effects and addiction, many countries prohibit their use unless prescribed by a physician, but they are often taken illegally. Page 150.

spiritual: relating to the soul or spirit, in contrast to material things. Page i.

spiritual gain: personal betterment in terms of an individual's own perceptions and abilities. Page 27.

spoiling: becoming rotten and unfit to eat because of decay. Page 13.

sponging: washing the body with a wet cloth or sponge. Page 41.

stable: firmly established; solid; fixed. Stable derives from Latin *stabilis,* meaning firm, steady. Page 1.

stagnant: lacking motion; not flowing or moving; inactive. Page 37.

stake, at: in danger of being lost. Page 95.

stamina: enduring physical energy and strength that allows somebody to do something for a long time. Page 168.

stampede: a sudden, headlong running away of a group of frightened animals, especially cattle or horses. Page 168.

standard: 1. precisely in accordance with the instructions and specifications for administering the Purification Program. Page 73.

2. demonstrating or accepted as normal or routine. Page 160.

startling: creating sudden surprise or wonder; astonishing. Page 19.

stem from: occur as a result of. Page 41.

steroids, (anabolic): drugs that promote muscle and bone growth (from *anabolism,* the process in the body of building body tissues). Steroids are used in medicine to promote healing, but when used for nonmedical purposes by athletes to temporarily increase the size of their muscles, these drugs are considered dangerous and are banned. Page 149.

stick to: continue something without giving up or abandoning it. Page 77.

stimulant(s): anything that temporarily increases the activity of some vital process or of some organ—specifically any food, beverage or other agent that temporarily increases the activity of such a process or organ. Page 9.

stimulate: cause physical activity in something, such as a nerve or an organ. Page 10.

Stoddard Solvent: a common *solvent,* a chemical substance that can dissolve other substances and is used to clean off oil, grease, paint, etc., from surfaces. Until the 1950s, it was also used in dry-cleaning processes. Named after W. J. Stoddard, who introduced it as a dry-cleaning fluid in the 1920s. Stoddard

Solvent poisoning is caused by swallowing or touching the solvent. Page 155.

stoned: being under the influence of a drug; drugged. Page 147.

strenuous: requiring or characterized by great effort or energy. Page 33.

stringently: (of regulations or procedures) strictly controlled by rule or standard; not loose; rigidly. Page 23.

subjected (to): made to undergo or experience (something unpleasant). Page 7.

subside: become less intense. Page 41.

subtle: slight and not very obvious. Page 168.

such and so: something not specified or not requiring to be specified. Page 107.

suds: a froth of bubbles on the surface of soapy water. Page 100.

sufficient: enough for a particular purpose; as much as one needs. Page 40.

supplant: replace (one thing) by something else. Page i.

supplement: (said of one's diet) improve by adding one or more substances with a particular nutritional value to make up for a deficiency. Page 23.

supplement(s): 1. a thing that is added to something else to improve or complete it, such as vitamin supplements taken in addition to what one usually eats. Page 61.

2. a part added to a book to supply additional information. Page 95.

suppressed: squashed; prevented from operating; restrained or limited in its effect. Page 71.

sweat-out: the action of releasing and eliminating impurities from the body while in a sauna or the period of time in which this is done. Page 23.

syndrome: the pattern of symptoms that characterize or indicate a particular condition. Page 166.

system: the entire human body considered as a functioning unit, as in *"apparently stays in the system."* Page 20.

take: a personal impression of, or response to, something, as in *"a fresh take on life."* Page 160.

take on: assume or acquire. Page 72.

taking place: happening or occurring. Page 80.

tandem, in: in association or partnership. Page 66.

tear gas: a gas that irritates the eyes severely, causing them to water and thus producing temporary blindness, used by the police or others, as in controlling riots. Page 159.

technology: the methods of application of an art or science as opposed to mere knowledge of the science or art itself. In Scientology, the term *technology* refers to the methods of application of Scientology principles to improve the functions of the mind and rehabilitate the potentials of the spirit, developed by L. Ron Hubbard. Page i.

tend: be generally inclined or likely to react or behave in a particular way; be in the habit of doing something. Page 72.

testimonials: written statements as to the value, excellence, etc., of a thing or that serve as evidence. Page 145.

Thorazine: a brand of *chlorpromazine,* a chemical substance used in psychiatry as a major tranquilizer. Thorazine is given to psychiatric patients to heavily sedate them as a supposed treatment for psychosis. Page 11.

three-dimensional: having, or seeming to have, the three measurable extents (dimensions) of height, width and depth. A cube is three-dimensional and a square is two-dimensional, having only height and width. Page 24.

thus: 1. therefore; as a consequence of. Page 1.

　　2. in this way or in the way just indicated. Page 23.

thus far: up to this point. Page 78.

time track: the consecutive record of mental image pictures which accumulates through a person's life. Page 24.

tissue(s): organic body material in humans, animals and plants made up of large numbers of cells that are similar in form and function. The four basic types of tissue are nerve, muscle, skin and connective (which support and hold parts of the body together). Page 20.

tolerance: (of the body) the ability to absorb a substance (such as a vitamin) continuously or in large doses. Page 123.

torturer: one who causes somebody severe pain to punish them or make them say or do something. Page 115.

toxic: poisonous or harmful to an organism. Page 1.

toxic mold: *mold* is a furry-type of growth on the surface of animal or vegetable matter, especially in the presence of dampness or decay. When present in very high quantities, some molds can bring about allergic reactions and are therefore considered toxic. Page 156.

toxin(s): originally, a poison produced by a living organism, which is capable of causing disease. The word later came to refer to any substance said to accumulate in the body, which is considered harmful or poisonous to the system. Page 8.

trace mineral(s): those minerals that have been found essential to maintaining life, found in the body in very small, i.e., *trace* amounts. Page 48.

tracking: following and understanding what is going on around one. Page 99.

tragedy(ies): a disastrous circumstance or event, such as serious illness, financial ruin or death. Page 100.

tranquilizer(s): any of certain drugs given as a supposed calming agent in controlling various emotional conditions. Page 7.

travails: pains, extreme anxieties or emotional torments or sufferings resulting from mental or physical hardship. Page 95.

"trip(s)": an experience undergone by someone taking drugs such as LSD or any similar drug. A "trip" can involve a range of sensations from mild to intense and often consists of euphoria (a false feeling of elation) and hallucination (the perception of objects with no reality and the experiencing of sensations without any external cause). These experiences can also occur to someone who took drugs in the past, even without taking them in the present. Page 20.

trustworthy: able to be relied on to be good, honest, sincere, etc. Page 108.

tuned in: sensitive to and aware of (something). Page 148.

turn on: cause to start operating or appear, as if by means of a switch, button or valve; activate. Page 53.

turpentine: a colorless, flammable, strong-smelling, bitter-tasting oil used as a paint solvent. Page 157.

twin: the partner with whom one is paired on the Purification Program. *Twin* means two similar, closely associated or otherwise paired persons, topics or objects. Page 40.

Tylenol: a brand name of a drug that is used in medicine to relieve pain and reduce fever. Page 154.

ultimate: 1. most extreme. Page 11.

2. lying beyond all others; forming the final aim or object. Page 80.

unaccustomed: not usual; unfamiliar. Page 49.

unbearable: too painful, annoying or unpleasant to deal with or accept. Page 99.

undertake: begin; enter upon. Page i.

uniform: always the same; not varying or changing in form, rate, degree, manner, etc.; constant. Page 107.

unique: being the only one of its kind. Page 28.

unleash: set something free as if from a leash or other form of restraint or confinement. Page 53.

unrelenting: not easing or lessening in strength, speed or effort. Page 12.

upbeat: positive and enthusiastic; feeling that the future will be good. Page 79.

upper atmosphere: the part of the atmosphere (mixture of gases surrounding the Earth) lying higher than the most immediate layer, that is, the atmosphere beyond 10 miles (16 kilometers) above the surface of the Earth. Page 14.

Valium: an addictive tranquilizing drug often prescribed by doctors or psychiatrists to "relieve" anxiety or tension. Page 11.

vast: very great in extent or degree. Page 7.

vein(s): any of the tubes that carry blood from all parts of the body to the heart. Page 66.

versus: as compared to or as one of two choices. Page 38.

vibrant: 1. dazzling or radiantly bright. Page 148.

    2. full of vigor and energy. Page 167.

vigor: energy, force or enthusiasm. Page 22.

vinyl paint: a paint that is made from a form of vinyl (any of various typically tough, flexible, shiny plastics). Page 69.

viral: of, pertaining to, or caused by a *virus*, a submicroscopic infectious agent that is twenty to one hundred times smaller than bacteria and which cannot survive outside of another living organism and must live in the cell of another living thing. Some viruses infect human beings with such diseases as measles, influenza and the common cold, others infect animals or plants, and still others even attack bacteria. Page 47.

vitality: great energy and liveliness; a large amount of physical and mental energy, usually combined with a wholehearted and joyous approach to situations and activities. Page 22.

vitamin: any of a group of substances that are used, in small amounts, for the normal functioning of the body. Vitamins are used by the body to help metabolize food (break down food in the body by chemical activity to produce the materials and energy necessary for life), to protect health and to aid in proper growth. Of the thirteen vitamins, five are produced by the body itself. The remaining need to be supplied through a person's daily diet. Page 1.

vitamin A: a vitamin found in some yellow and dark-green vegetables, and also animal products such as egg yolk, milk and fish-liver oils. Vitamin A aids in the health of the outer layer of cells in the skin and organs. Page 125.

vitamin B complex: a group of water-soluble vitamins found in yeast, eggs, liver and vegetables, essential in normal body growth and nerve function. Page 70.

vitamin B$_1$: a vitamin found in green peas, beans, egg yolks, liver and the outer coating of cereal grains. It assists in the absorption of carbohydrates and enables carbohydrates to release the energy required for cellular function. A *carbohydrate* is one of the three main classes of food (the others are fats and protein) that provide energy to the body. Page 11.

vitamin C: a water-soluble vitamin found in citrus fruits, tomatoes, raw onions, raw potatoes and leafy green vegetables. It helps promote healthy gums and teeth, aids in mineral absorption, helps heal wounds and aids the prevention and treatment of the common cold. Vitamin C reacts with any foreign substance reaching the blood and helps to detoxify the system and prevent toxic reactions caused by drugs. Page 45.

vitamin D: a vitamin found in such foods as egg yolks and liver, and manufactured by the body in the skin through exposure to sunlight. Vitamin D enables the body to absorb and use *calcium,* a mineral vital to the health of bones and teeth. Page 125.

vitamin E: a vitamin naturally occurring in vegetable oils, butter, eggs, cereal grains and leafy green vegetables. Vitamin E plays a role in forming red blood cells, muscle and other tissues and is important for fertility in humans. Page 125.

vitamin therapy: the use of nutrition to decrease the incidence of disease or symptoms. Page 1.

volume: a large quantity or amount of something. Page 8.

vying: competing strongly in order to obtain or achieve something. Page 9.

waste(s): an unwanted or unusable byproduct of something, such as radiation. Page 8.

wear off: gradually disappear or stop. Page 108.

weigh (something) against: assess the relative importance of (one thing in relation to another). Page 103.

well-being: general health and happiness. Page 1.

whamo: a term used to signify startling action, change, etc. Page 168.

whatsoever: of any kind at all. Used to emphasize a negative statement, after words such as no, none, no one, etc. Page 160.

wheat rust: a fungus that attacks the roots of wheat plants and produces reddish marks on the stems and leaves. Page 20.

whereof: of what, which or whom. Page 45.

wholesale: in large quantities. Page 45.

wholly: completely, entirely or thoroughly. Page 72.

widespread: existing or happening over a large area or among many people. Page 1.

will: a legal document containing a statement of what somebody wants to have happen to his or her property after he or she dies. Page 160.

winded: unable to breathe in enough air easily; short of breath. Page 165.

win(s): an accomplishment of any desired improvement. Examples of wins would be a person experiencing an increased feeling of well-being or gaining more certainty about some area of his life. Page 149.

withdrawal: a period during which somebody addicted to a drug stops taking it, causing the person to experience painful physical and mental reactions known as withdrawal symptoms. Page i.

wooden(ness): without spirit, animation or awareness; also, dull or stupid. Page 108.

worked up: developed or produced by physical effort. Page 39.

World Trade Center (WTC): a complex in New York City that included twin skyscrapers (the tallest in the US at 110 stories). These buildings were destroyed on September 11 (9/11), 2001, when two jetliners, hijacked by terrorists, were flown into them, causing the worst building disaster in recorded history and the deaths of some 2,800 people. Page 163.

wreak havoc: cause or produce harm, damage, etc. Page 8.

wretched: extremely bad or unpleasant; miserable. Page 115.

wrought: brought about or caused by. Page 2.

X-rays: invisible waves consisting of tiny particles of energy that are able to go through soft materials in the same way light passes through glass. When this occurs, energy is transferred to the material and damage can result. They are called *X-rays* as, at the time of their discovery, they were rays of unknown origin. They are commonly used by hospitals and doctors to show pictures of the inside of the body. Page 15.

zest: great enthusiasm, liveliness or energy. Page 146.

zinc: a mineral that is vital to many biological functions such as immune resistance, wound healing, digestion, reproduction, physical growth, taste and smell. The body needs zinc to make good use of vitamin A. Page 126.

$\mathcal{I}$NDEX

anesthetics, 69

restimulation of, 40

arsenic, 10

artificial sweeteners, 13

asbestos products

workers in factories that
produce or use, 12

aspirin

addicts, 108

mental image pictures
and, 108

painkiller, 107

what the compulsion
to take aspirin stems
from, 108

asthma, 152, 154, 164

atmosphere

deterioration of upper, 14

atomic power, 14

B

biochemical

definition, 7

biochemistry, 45

painkillers and, 107

biophysical handlings, 27

life-hostile elements
and, 27

Bioplasma

cell salts, 41

blankness

drugs and, 27, 99

pain depressants and, 108

body

composed of, 8

disarranging of
biochemistry and fluid
balance of, 22

reconstructing after
drugs, 89

body odors

sweating out impurities, 71

B$_1$, *see* vitamin B$_1$

brain

marijuana and atrophy
of, 10

bronchial symptoms

turning on and
vanishing, 70

C

caffeine

drug, 9

calcium

acidic base and, 66

basic building block, 65

creating vitamin C
deficiency and, 48

importance of, 65

mistakes and, 100

most destructive element in current culture, 10

not used on Purification Program, i

out of present time and, 99

perceiving something else going on, 100

perceptions distorted by, 24

person not running in the same series of events as others, 100

procreation before death and, 95

psychiatric, *see* **psychiatric drugs**

reconstructing body after, 89

remove a person from present time, 99

research of effect on body, mind and spirit, 2

residuals, in body for years, 47

restimulation and, 40

twin and, 40

schools employing, 103

sexual stimulation and, 95

street, *see* **street drugs**

sweating out, 21, 22

trap, 1

unrealities and, 99

vitamin B$_1$, burning up, 117

vitamin burn-up and, 45

wearing off and ability to create mental image pictures, 108

withdrawal symptoms and, 115

workers in factories that produce, 12

see also **medicine**

D.T.'s, 46

dullness

going through a period of, 71

dyes

workers in factories that produce or use, 12

E

education

impeded by drugs, 103–104

psychiatric drugs impeding, 103

electrical equipment

workers in factories that produce, 12

elemental

definition, 131

emotions

reappearance of, 71

endocrine system

drugs upsetting, 48

minerals and trace minerals and, 48

End Phenomena

niacin and, 127

Purification Program, 85

"enhancers," 13

environment

life-hostile elements in, 8

essential fatty acids

definition, 61

ethical fiber

drugs and breakdown of, 11

evening primrose oil

use of, 141

exercise

after program completion, 127

sauna and, 37

F

fainting

heat exhaustion and, 41

fat

difficulty metabolizing, 141

evening primrose oil and, 141

middle age and breaking down, 20

trading bad fat for good oil, 60

illustration, 60

see also **fatty tissue**

fatty acids

definition, 61

essential

definition, 61

fatty tissue

LSD lodging in, 20

middle age and breaking down, 20

toxic substances locking up in, 59, 61

see also **fat**

fearful condition

niacin and, 55

fertilizers

man-made, 13

workers in factories that produce or use, 12

flashbacks

LSD, 21, 69

floor

cleaning the floor, example of alteration by someone on drugs, 100

O

THINK CLEARLY

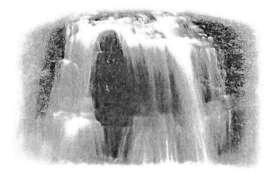

How do drugs and toxins affect your everyday life?

These substances can lodge in your body for years, dulling your perceptions and dimming your awareness—even destroying your life.

The solution: L. Ron Hubbard's Purification Program.

Like a fresh stream of crystal-clear water, it eliminates the effects of the harmful substances that block your clear thinking—restoring *life* and *vitality*.

Tens of thousands around the world say they are living happier, more successful lives today as a result of the Purification Program. It can do the same for *you*.

DO THE

PURIFICATION PROGRAM